IMMUNIZATION

Everything You Need to Know About Vaccinations
and Immune-Boosting Therapies for Your Child

Harriet Griffey

E L E M E N T

Shaftesbury, Dorset • Boston, Massachusetts • Melbourne, Victoria

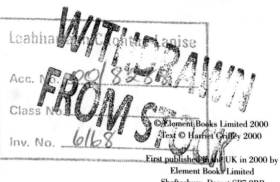

© Element Books Limited 2000
Text © Harriet Griffey 2000

First published in the UK in 2000 by
Element Books Limited
Shaftesbury, Dorset SP7 8BP

Published in the US in 2000 by
Element Books, Inc
160 North Washington Street
Boston, MA 02114

Published in Australia in 2000 by
Element Books and distributed by
Penguin Australia Limited
487 Maroondah Highway, Ringwood,
Victoria 3134

Cover design by:
THE BRIDGEWATER BOOK COMPANY
Design and Typeset by:
THE BRIDGEWATER BOOK COMPANY
Printed and bound in Great Britain by Creative Print and Design, Ebbw Vale, Wales

British Library Cataloguing in Publication data available

Library of Congress Cataloging in Publication data available

ISBN 1 86204 541 0

Contents

For my children, Josh and Robbie.

Introduction

The debate about whether or not to routinely immunize children against previously common childhood illnesses has gained momentum over recent years, making it increasingly difficult for parents to determine what's best for their children. It is a subject which challenges aspects of what it means to be a parent in today's world. We will be judged by what we do and what we don't do, whether we immunize our children or whether we don't, and by our views on social responsibility to those children who, for one reason or another, cannot be immunized. Parenting is no easy task.

When I began researching this book, I wanted to look at immunization within the context of promoting the positive health of a child, providing information which would help parents make choices about various aspects of healthcare, including whether or not to immunize. And as I continued looking into the masses of research material available, I became increasingly aware of how polarized the debate has become, and how unhelpful this is for the majority of parents. On the one hand, health authorities are unequivocal that immunization is best, and on the other, the anti-immunization lobby is adamant that it is, at best, to be avoided and, at worst, a conspiratorial plot to exert statutory control over a population of children. But even if you explore both sides of the argument with great care, you are still left with the parents' dilemma: you still have to make a decision. And for many, making an objective decision about such a subjective matter as whether or not to give a healthy child an injection with the potential, however remote, that it might make them ill, is very difficult. So we do the best we can and make decisions based on what we believe to be right for each individual child.

That the debate exists at all is important, and the Department of Health in the UK, for example, is well aware of parental anxieties and concern about immunization. The fact that doctors receive payments linked to the percentage of children immunized, and how this policy is interpreted by parents, cannot be ignored. To those parents who feel they are being coerced into having their children immunized, it looks as though doctors might be putting profit before children's health. But wherever there is debate there is also continuing pressure to ensure that research, monitoring, assessment and reporting are carried out with greater effectiveness, and that can only be a good thing.

Opposition to immunization isn't new, it began with immunization itself and has continued over the last 200 years. In the UK an anti-vaccination lobby existed in the early 1800s in response to Jenner's discovery of the smallpox vaccine, and it wasn't until 1948 that legislation enforcing vaccination was finally withdrawn. The idea of compulsory vaccination seems draconian today, but in an attempt to reduce the incidence of disease, it was once thought an appropriate measure. In the US, although not compulsory, immunization remains a necessity for school entry. Except on ideological or religious grounds – but not often on medical grounds – all children are expected to be immunized, although this policy is often interpreted at state level.

Your view of this debate depends in part on your personal point of view: on whether you consider vaccination as merely one of several preventative health measures available to us – along with, for example, cervical smear tests, glaucoma testing and mammography – or as a thinly-disguised plot to save money on the health budget and line the pockets of drug companies. Like any preventative health measure, vaccination is not foolproof, and perhaps the greatest disservice that the routine immunization programme has done over the last 30 years is to suggest that this is all that is required to ensure children's good health. If chosen, immunization can only ever be one of several steps parents take to protect the health of their children.

Vaccination exists only because the possibility of creating immunity without having the illness was discovered in the first place. Wherever there is a virus, there exists this possibility. So research often looks for a viral cause for illnesses like cancer or Alzheimer's disease in order to try and find a cure, based on what has been learnt about preventative health measures from the development of immunization. The possibility of a vaccine for Alzheimer's disease 'within the next five years' (according to researchers in July 1999) would be heralded as a considerable breakthrough, for example.

For those generations that lived in fear of polio, the arguments against immunization hardly exist. For later generations, pictures from the 1950s of rows and rows of people in iron lungs – which they needed in order to breathe because their diaphragms were paralysed by the disease – carry little weight: we know we are protected, both by improved sanitation and by immunization. To most people the spectre of congenital rubella syndrome no longer exists; German measles has declined to the point where we believe the risk to be so small that we even consider not having our children immunized. And smallpox, which gave rise to the first immunization in 1796, has declined to such a degree that immunization is no longer necessary. And this may, in turn, be the case for other illnesses, polio for example. But it wasn't always so. Parents were once as frightened of polio as we are today of meningitis. This fear can be demonstrated by the demand for vaccination every time a possible outbreak of meningitis is heralded by the death of a child. When a risk becomes that close, few people want to take it.

In the UK, a new vaccination for meningitis C was introduced in the autumn of 1999, much to the relief of many parents. In the previous year there had been around 2,600 cases, double the number in 1988, and around 10 per cent of the children affected had died, while around one third of survivors were left permanently disabled in some way. But doctors warn against a false sense of security: meningitis B, the form of the disease responsible for around 60 per cent of cases in the UK (although fewer result in deaths), still has no vaccine. Parents cannot be complacent and rely on immunization; they have to remain vigilant and care for their children's health in a variety of ways, of which immunization may only be one.

There is no doubt that as medical science advances, expectations rise. For instance, if a nation has the wherewithal, we expect it to be used to safeguard the health of the population. And if doctors had this capacity but didn't use it to the benefit of the people, this would certainly be questioned. Indeed, this occurs when we look at developing countries and ask why, for example, there are still so many children crippled by polio, placing an enormous burden on their families, communities and the country as a whole, when we know how to reduce the impact of this disease and developed countries have benefited from this knowledge for years.

Many of today's parents, however, can see no reason for routine vaccination against diseases which don't appear to exist. Some parents are quite strongly opposed to immunization against illnesses that pose no apparent threat. We can all rest assured that the risk of catching diphtheria in the UK, even if we have not been immunized, is virtually non-existent (one death in 1994, in an unimmunized child who had caught it in Pakistan). It's difficult to see these risks in the abstract, even when we are told that when immunization levels drop within a community the risk reappears. For example, after the immunization scheme in Russia collapsed, there were 52,000 cases of diphtheria in 1995 and 1,700 people died. Sweden phased out its routine immunization for whooping cough in 1979, but the incidence increased and resulted in two outbreaks in 1983 and 1985, with some deaths associated with complications. Immunization there has now been reintroduced.

Trying to assess risk, and in particular the risk of contracting an illness for which there appears to be no incidence, and the comparative risks associated with immunization, is undoubtedly difficult. Even if research were to show that in a particular illness the risk of developing a complication was 1,000 times higher than the risk of that same complication arising from immunization, to those who don't believe there is a risk of that illness in the first place, the difference between the two risks would be immaterial. But even if the risk is only 1 in 1,000, it is still a risk: you may be the 1 in 1,000 who is affected.

And of course there is the recognizable risk to a child's health through being vaccinated, as is evident from the UK's Vaccine Damage Payments Act of 1979. Vaccine damage is difficult to prove, but there have been successful cases, and payments have been made, although many other claims of damage remain unproven. As a consequence, in the UK a number of groups have formed: JABS (Justice, Awareness and Basic Support), the Vaccination Awareness Network UK, The Informed Parent, and What the Doctors Don't Tell You. They all provide a powerful counter-resource to material provided by the UK Department of Health, and are definitely anti-vaccination.

The arguments for and against vaccination are not easy. While one source stresses a link between MS and measles, another suggests that measles immunization might be the cause of Crohn's disease. And for every piece of research suggesting a causative link between immunization and a health disorder, another shows none. For example, while one source claims a definitive link between immunization and cot death, an equally reputable source says there is no link.

It seems increasingly clear that a range of external influences to which babies and young children are exposed, including immunization, may trigger an unexpected response. It remains a deeply unsettling fact that we just don't know the consequences of some of the decisions we make on behalf of our children. But decision making, however difficult, lies at the heart of parenting.

We have become, over the years, increasingly keen to identify cause and effect, so when a health problem arises we automatically look for a cause. In turn this has led to more specific diagnoses and treatments. For example, many reasons are given for the increased number of asthma cases diagnosed – central heating; environmental pollution; an excess of milk, wheat and sugar in the diet; childhood vaccination; the desire of drug companies to boost profits; a lack of environmental dirt. These are all explanations that can be backed up by research, but which conclusion is correct?

There is also concern about the long-term damage immunization might do. Dr Michel Odent, the eminent obstetrician who runs the Primal Health Research Centre in the UK, has been monitoring research which suggests that immunization is linked to increased rates of asthma in children. Professor Graham Rook, an immunologist at University College, London, has convincing research to show that an absence of dirt (and the micro-organisms it contains) in their daily life restricts children from receiving the immune stimulus they need to 'switch on' those cells that work to prevent the development of allergies. Although vaccination can 'switch on' one sort of immunity, this needs to be balanced by the stimulation needed to protect children against allergies. While improved hygiene and sanitation may be a general improvement, we obviously need other stimuli in order to develop a truly effective immune system.

In alternative practices, and in Traditional Chinese medicine in particular, there is a view that children need to experience acute eruptive infections, like measles, in order to shake off toxins and create an internally strong immune system, which in turn will lead to good health. It is also thought that childhood infections help off-load toxins that a child is born with, having inherited them from its parents. Alternative practitioners believe that gaining immunity through immunization is not as effective as experiencing the active eruption of the illness. However, should you decide against immunization and your child does catch a life-threatening illness – measles, for example – it is essential that you are able to take the necessary time to look after your child and allow him or her to recover adequately, otherwise the illness can be a terrible drain on the child's health and immune system.

Over the years, our attitude to early childhood illnesses has changed: we no longer expect our children to be ill, nor do we have the lifestyles to support looking after a sick child for up to two weeks at a time. If you look in the numerous childcare manuals available for today's parents, there is little information included about looking after sick children. Those illnesses of childhood once described as common are no longer so.

And yet children continue to be unwell, even if in less tangible ways than having a full-blown case of the measles. According to a British Medical Association report published in

July 1999, children in Britain are among the least healthy in Europe, putting Britain at number 18 out of the top 20 nations featured in the report. The report was based on the child mortality rate, i.e. the number of deaths under five years of age per 1,000 live births. In Britain the number of deaths per 1,000 is seven, whereas in Sweden, Singapore and Finland it is four, and in Slovenia, Japan, France, Monaco, Iceland and Australia, five. Britain's higher figure has been attributed largely to its widening poverty gap, with children under five in the lowest income level four times more likely to die of an accident than those in the highest income level, and nearly twice as likely to suffer long-standing illnesses. Nutrition is often poor, with 1 in 12 British children between the age of 18 months and five years suffering from iron-deficiency anaemia.

This brings me back to one of the aims of this book: to provide not only information on immunization, but also a context where immunization is but one of several options to consider in regard to children's health, along with diet, exercise, sleep and the use of alternative and complementary therapies. We cannot have it both ways. We cannot fully immunize our children and then neglect other ways of promoting positive health. And if we choose to reject immunization, we must realize that children, however healthy, may still be at risk if they haven't been able to acquire immunity through illness. There are options and choices, but, as with many other aspects of parenting, there are no certainties.

1

The Immune System

We are all born with our immune system in place, but the development of immunity occurs in response to exposure to those micro-organisms that can cause illness and disease. The process begins at birth, but because the immune system needs to develop over time, newborns are quite vulnerable. They rely initially on the protection provided by passive immunity – in antibodies received from the mother before birth – and the antibodies and anti-infective agents in breastmilk. But the actual development of immunity needs to be triggered by exposure, after birth, to those bugs that will make a child's body produce its own antibodies.

Most of us have some idea of what the immune system is and roughly how it works, but it is worth thinking about it a little more fully when considering how babies grow and develop, and how we can promote the positive health of our children. Our general health is influenced by many factors, not least by our genes, about which we can do little, but also by diet and lifestyle, which we do have some control over. This book looks at ways to promote a lifestyle that can support the development of a child's immunity. This includes both exposure to microorganisms, and, if appropriate, immunization.

The ability of the immune system to recognize substances that are 'foreign' and potentially damaging is the key to how it works. However, it is possible to develop immunity to some micro-organisms without suffering a full-blown bout of illness, and when this happens it is described as being 'sub-clinical', i.e. there are no apparent clinical symptoms of the illness. For example, as adults the number of cold viruses we are exposed to is far greater than the number of colds we experience. This is not necessarily because we have an immunity to that particular virus – there are too many variations for that to be likely – but because our body is used to being exposed to cold viruses in general and responds quickly to produce antibodies. On the occasions when we are, for a number of reasons, 'below par', then we might succumb to the symptoms of a cold – sore throat, fever, runny nose – which may last for up to five days, the life of the virus itself. Colds often seem to happen at times of stress, or immediately after, as if the body has given itself permission to 'let go', which suggests quite clearly that the mind/body link is relevant to our health.

In infants and children, the gradual exposure to bacteria and to viruses like the common cold helps develop immunity. So while children may appear to be more susceptible, getting a cold is in fact part of a necessary process. During a time of illness, however, it is important that a child receives adequate rest and nutrition to support the body, enable recovery and help build further immunity.

However, a baby's immune system needs time to mature and if it is overloaded, or exposed to an excess of viruses or bacteria, this can be detrimental. Certainly during the first few months of life it is worth taking a few sensible precautions, such as asking visitors to wash their hands before handling your baby, or tactfully asking those with coughs and colds to stay away. Equally, communal childcare before the age of three is often thought to be inadvisable because of the excessive number of viruses and bacteria to which a child can be exposed.

Research has indicated that children in larger families are less prone to full-blown disease because they are generally exposed to more bugs at an early age and are therefore able to build up immunity. Close family members and siblings who are in regular contact with you and your baby are thus not such a risk, especially if you are breastfeeding, because the benefits of antibodies and anti-infective agents present in breastmilk help protect your baby while immunity is developing – as will the passive immunity during the first year of life. However, the hand-washing rule is still a useful one to apply, especially with siblings! Soap and water alone are quite adequate; there's no need to use antibacterial handwashes which can actually destroy 'friendly' bacteria that co-exist happily on our skin and serve a useful purpose.

The immune system is quite complicated to understand, but it's worth considering how it works and in particular how it works in conjunction with the other defence systems of the body.

The body's defence systems

The immune system forms part of the body's defence system against the harm and damage that can be caused by the outside world. Although the way it functions is extremely important it is but one of three lines of defence, together with mechanical barriers (e.g. the skin) and inflammatory responses.

Mechanical barriers

One of the primary forms of protection we have against disease and illness is the skin, which forms a physical barrier to protect against potentially damaging germs. A slightly oily barrier is produced by the secretions of the sebaceous glands, and a natural antiseptic in the secretions from the sweat glands also helps. In addition, the skin's surface naturally plays host to a number of bacteria which help prevent more damaging germs gaining access. These 'friendly' bacteria 'eat up' harmful substances, so their presence is beneficial and, unless the balance is disturbed, do no harm.

All the body passages that open onto the skin surface, for example the nose, are lined with a mucous membrane, which also has a protective function. The mucus produced by the cells of the mucosal membrane helps to trap germs and discourages their further entry into the body. In the nose and upper respiratory tract there are also tiny hairs called cilia which move the secreted mucus, with any trapped germs, forward to the outside, thus assisting its removal from the body. Eyes are protected by the production of tears, which contain an antibacterial substance called lysozyme, and the stomach produces hydrochloric acid, lethal to many of the bacteria swallowed. So although the body is subject to a daily bombardment of germs, it makes a supreme effort to see off most of them.

Inflammatory responses

Inflammation is the body's response to both injury and infection. First the small blood vessels around the area dilate, slowing down the flow of blood and causing a degree of redness and swelling. This also causes the pain often experienced, because the swelling presses on surrounding nerve endings. The blood supply allows a concentration of specialized white blood cells to do their job in breaking down the bacteria, diluting the toxins and forming a barrier to prevent their spread. The degree of activity that occurs will depend on whether or not there is an infection. If the bacterium has caused an infection before, and been recognized by the body as a trigger or antigen, then antibodies will be present to tackle the infection.

Our bodies are well adapted to share our environment with enormous numbers of micro-organisms, chemicals and other substances, and it is in part our continued exposure to potentially damaging substances that helps our body systems to mature and immunity to develop.

Immunity

The immune system consists of the organs in the body which respond to the presence of substances that are recognized as 'foreign'. This is why in the case of transplanted organs immuno-suppressive drugs have to be given to protect the new organ from rejection. Even pregnancy, where the growing baby is literally a foreign body, has an effect on the immune system, suppressing it so that the fetus is not rejected.

In most cases, however, foreign substances are what we loosely describe as 'germs' – bacteria, viruses, parasites, fungi – which can cause infection. When they are recognized by the immune system, an immune response is triggered. Anything that triggers the immune response is called an antigen.

The first time the immune system encounters a particular antigen, it takes some time to produce the antibodies which will render it harmless. And it is during this time that we may experience symptoms of the illness itself. Subsequently, however, infection by the same antigen will produce a much quicker response, making the germ harmless before it has time to do any damage. We then have immunity to that antigen – and in future only to an identical antigen: cold viruses, for example, come in many, many different forms so it isn't possible to become totally immune to the common cold.

Antibodies are proteins produced by lymphocytes (a type of white blood cell). These are produced by the lymph nodes, which are part of the lymphatic system that circulates throughout the body. During an infection swollen lymph nodes can sometimes be felt around the neck, or in the groin or armpit, and this swelling gives an indication that the immune system is working. Lymphocytes are also produced by the lymphoid tissue in the tonsils and adenoids, bone marrow, liver, spleen and thymus gland. Lymphocytes and antibodies constantly circulate in the blood and lymphatic system, ready to respond when needed.

The group of naturally occurring proteins that act as antibodies are known as immunoglobulins. There are five different types of antibody immunoglobulin – IgA, IgD, IgE, IgG and IgM – and they each have a different role to play. It is possible to measure the levels of antibodies in the blood; the HIV test, for example, measures the presence of antibodies to the human immunodeficiency virus (HIV) following an infection. What is not easy to judge is the level of antibody required to prevent reinfection by an antigen. While you may develop antibodies to a particular germ, you may not have enough to prevent reinfection. This explains why some people get chickenpox a second time, for example.

Passive immunity

During its last months in the womb, a baby receives antibodies to certain illnesses from its mother's blood, via the placenta. This provides a degree of immunity – known as passive immunity – to help protect the child during the first year of life. Some antibodies, for example those which protect against whooping cough, appear to offer little or no protection, but antibodies to measles, if they are present in the mother, may offer protection for 6 to 12 months. It is impossible to gauge how much protection is available to a baby through passive immunity, or how a baby would react to an infection should it occur. With premature babies there is a reduced level of protection, because antibodies are only transferred during the last months of pregnancy. This makes them more vulnerable than babies born at term.

Passive immunity can also be acquired through an injection of human immunoglobulin, which provides immediate protection although it lasts only a few weeks. Immunoglobulins for tetanus, hepatitis, rabies and chickenpox, for example, obtained from the pooled blood of convalescent patients, or donors who have been recently immunized, can be injected to provide short-term protection.

Active immunity

Active immunity is long term and can be induced by immunization, where a vaccine is given either by injection or, as with polio, by mouth. Vaccines may be attenuated, which means that they are live but weakened, or they may be dead, so either way they are unable to cause a full-blown illness but can stimulate antibodies and create immunity. The vaccine for measles, mumps and rubella (MMR), for example, contains attenuated viruses, while the standard whooping cough vaccine contains dead bacteria.

The body responds to the vaccine in the same way as it does to any antigen – it produces antibodies, as though it had been exposed to a natural infection – but does not develop the full-blown disease. As a result, immunity is acquired and because of the immune system's 'memory', next time there is any exposure to the same antigen, the immune system is already primed to fight off the disease. But an individual's reaction is just that – individual. While some people produce masses of antibodies to an infection of chickenpox, others don't. In the same way, some produce masses of antibodies in response to immunization, while others don't. Is it therefore difficult to ascertain who is adequately protected – either by immunization or by a previous occurrence of the disease – and who isn't.

In most Western countries a childhood immunization programme will offer vaccinations for diphtheria, tetanus and pertussis (whooping cough), or DTP; polio; *Haemophilus influenzae* type B (Hib); and measles, mumps and rubella (MMR). Vaccination against tuberculosis (BCG) is offered at around 13 years of age.

Herd immunity

When the majority of the population is immunized against a particular disease, the incidence of that disease in the community is reduced. This reduced incidence also helps to protect those members of the community who can't, for whatever reason, be immunized against the disease. Those for whom vaccination would be dangerous – the very young, the very old, and those suffering from immuno-suppressive illness – thus benefit from the protection of herd immunity because the overall risk of infection is reduced.

However, because it can never be known what percentage of those immunized will produce adequate, protective antibodies, any immunization programme requires a certain uptake to protect those who cannot develop immunity or have not yet done so. Further, no vaccine is 100 per cent effective, so if the percentage of the immunized population falls below a certain level, herd immunity is reduced.

A reduced response to immunization can be useful in reducing the severity of a disease, even if it doesn't wholly prevent infection. For example, one survey showed that of 8,000 children vaccinated against whooping cough, a few still got the disease – but in a much less severe form. In general, even when vaccination 'fails' it is found to reduce the severity of the disease.

What has to be understood about the immune system is that it can only protect against diseases to which it has been previously exposed, in one form or another. However fit and healthy you are, and however able you are to deal with illness, your immune system cannot prevent you from getting a disease from which you have no immunity. Good health in itself isn't protection enough, although it will help the body to respond and adequately cope with illness.

There is also the danger that a period of reduced immunity of several weeks or longer following an infection (measles, for example) can make a child vulnerable to other illness. So although a child may recover well from a disease, that disease may have compromised the immune system in general and increased the risk of subsequent infections.

While it is true that in malnourished populations, serious illness and death are associated with infectious diseases, it is difficult to say for certain that there is a direct link between malnutrition and low immunity because overcrowding, poverty and poor sanitation are also important factors. And in the same way, it isn't possible to say for certain that improved nutrition and housing alone have brought about a reduction in infectious diseases in developed countries, because the contribution of vaccines must also be considered.

2

Childhood immunization

Immunity and immunization is a huge subject, and one around which there is much debate. However, in order to make choices, information is needed about the role played by immunization in the acquisition of active immunity: i.e. a state which enables the body to produce its own antibodies. The purpose of this chapter is to cover some essential aspects of immunization and provide a basis on which you can find out whether or not immunization is relevant or important to your child.

There are two ways to acquire immunity to an illness: having the disease itself, and being immunized. Immunization consists of a dose of dead or weakened virus or bacteria being injected into the body (except for polio vaccine, which is usually taken by mouth). A vaccine is designed to stimulate the body to produce antibodies, but it is not strong enough to cause an infection of the actual disease.

Smallpox – a case history

The history of immunization – or vaccination, or inoculation – began in the UK in 1796 when a doctor, Edward Jenner, discovered that dairymaids who caught cowpox seemed immune to the devastating disease of smallpox. He then injected the contents of a cowpox pustule into an eight-year-old boy, who became ill with the non-life-threatening cowpox. Once the boy had recovered, Jenner injected him with smallpox. The illness didn't occur because the boy's first injection of cowpox had created immunity to smallpox, as Jenner correctly surmised.

This rather unethical experiment worked, and the idea of immunization was introduced. At the time, very few people reached adulthood without catching smallpox, and 10 per cent of people died from it. At the end of the 18th century, smallpox caused one fifth of all deaths in Glasgow, and nine out of ten people who died of smallpox were under the age of five.

From the start the debate about vaccination was active, as was the anti-vaccination lobby. In the UK the Vaccination Acts of 1840, 1841 and 1853 actively encouraged vaccination by making it universally free, and in successive Acts of 1861, 1867 and 1871 it was made compulsory. It continued to be so until 1948, when the compulsory Vaccination Act was repealed.

The last UK epidemic of smallpox was in London in 1901, and the world's last naturally occurring case was in 1977 in Somalia. However, by the mid-1970s, 175 years after it was introduced, smallpox vaccination was no longer considered necessary for protection against the disease because, effectively, smallpox no longer existed. In May 1980, the World Health Assembly declared that, because of the success of the global programme of vaccination, smallpox had been eradicated.

Production of vaccines

The vaccines given to children divide into four main categories: those containing live, but weakened viruses (for example, MMR for measles, mumps and rubella, and Sabin, an oral polio vaccine); dead, complete bacteria (for example, whooping cough vaccine); inactivated bacterial toxins (for example, tetanus and diphtheria vaccine); and purified bacterial sugars (for example, Hib vaccine).

Live vaccines are grown in different ways. The measles and mumps components of the MMR vaccine are grown in cell cultures from chicken's eggs, which is why anyone with an extreme reaction to egg proteins should be assessed carefully and only given the MMR vaccine under close supervision. The rubella vaccines are grown in a cell culture called MRC5, which was originally developed from a small number of cells from a fetus aborted for medical reasons in the 1960s, and the manufacturing process removes all traces of the cells the vaccine was grown in.

Depending on the type and needs of the vaccine, the fluid in which it is given may be sterile water, sterile salt water or a necessary tissue culture fluid. Sometimes extremely small quantities of chemicals are needed to stabilize the vaccine, while many contain thiomersal, derived from mercury, to prevent contamination. Some vaccines also contain an aluminium compound, which is designed to improve the body's response to the vaccine. In rare cases, if someone is sensitive to these additives, an allergic reaction might occur.

Testing of vaccines

Unlike many other countries, the UK has a comprehensive and well-established system of monitoring the incidence of infectious diseases and of vaccine uptake. In contrast, in the US, no national information is collected on vaccine uptake and while proof of immunization for infectious diseases is needed in all states before children start school, parents can opt out of immunization on ideological or religious grounds. In Germany, there are no national statistics on vaccine uptake and although there is a national immunization policy, this is interpreted at a local level.

What the UK provides, as a consequence, is a useful model of how careful monitoring can help contribute to safety and effectiveness. The following information, although specific to the UK, provides an overview of the scrupulous attention to detail that needs to form the basis of any immunization programme.

UK procedures

Before a vaccine can be licensed for use, it has to undergo tests to prove its safety and effectiveness. These tests, or trials, are designed to assess three main aspects of a vaccine: the extent of antibody response, its effectiveness at protecting against the disease, and the type and frequency of any reactions. Trials of a new vaccine, and indeed of any new medicine, have to be carried out in three phases, each of which has to be passed before moving on to the next.

Phase 1

The vaccine is administered only to a small number of healthy adult volunteers, to check whether it causes any unexpected or serious side effects.

Phase 2

The vaccine is given to between 100 and 200 individuals within the category for which the vaccine is intended. Blood tests measure the antibody response, and the types of more common reactions and their frequency are recorded. These results are compared against a control group not receiving the vaccine. Where Phase 2 is carried out within a group of children, parents are asked to record information about side effects.

Phase 3

The number of vaccinated and unvaccinated people who get the disease is assessed. A vaccine is only considered effective if the incidence of disease in those who have been immunized is significantly lower than in those who did not receive the vaccine.

Only after these trials have been successfully completed is the product licensed for use. However, strict quality controls apply and every batch of vaccine produced has to be tested before it can be released to ensure that each dose will be safe and effective. Not only does the manufacturer have to carry out quality control and testing on every batch of vaccine but, in addition, so must an independent assessor.

Even after a vaccine has been licensed the testing and evaluation continues, monitoring for safety, any rare or new reactions, and its effectiveness in preventing illness. This is done in combination with monitoring the effectiveness of the immunization programme in general, through both surveillance of the disease and special surveys. Such vigilance can help to indicate when a change in vaccination policy might be necessary, or to predict that a population might be at risk of an outbreak of a particular disease.

In 1995, for example, surveys and studies showed that the number of children susceptible to measles rose between 1986 and 1991. Calculations based on this information indicated that the increased susceptibility of children increased the risk of an outbreak, or epidemic, of measles. The Department of Health therefore felt it necessary to take steps in order to avoid this possibility and initiated a mass immunization campaign in the November of that year to vaccinate schoolchildren against measles.

MONITORING ADVERSE SIDE EFFECTS

Monitoring and reporting on adverse side effects continue while a vaccine is in use. Health professionals are asked to report side effects and reactions to the Committee on Safety of Medicines. As a voluntary reporting system, it is not without problems, including under-reporting, no standard criteria for reporting, and no follow-up procedures. A new system is currently being explored where hospital admission records are linked with immunization records in order to pick up all possible connections where there is any evidence of side effects.

In the UK, as elsewhere, there is an enormous commitment to ensuring the safety and effectiveness of immunization, in spite of criticism that parents are being coerced into immunizing their children in order to fulfil doctors' quotas and ensure full remuneration from the Department of Health ... and to line the pockets of drug companies. But it is not really in anyone's interest to license for use a product that causes damage, so everything is done to ensure that a product is both safe and effective.

CHANGES IN IMMUNIZATION POLICIES

As described above, constant monitoring and surveillance can lead to occasional changes to immunization programme policies; for example, the smallpox vaccination is no longer deemed necessary. And in 1990, the schedule for the infant immunization programme was changed in the UK. Previously, the first schedule of immunizations for diphtheria, tetanus, whooping cough and polio started at three months and was completed at 10–11 months. Now it begins at two months and is completed at four months. The change was made in order to protect those most at risk from severe complications of whooping cough – babies under six months old, where 1 in 100 dies from complications. The whooping cough component is not now included in the pre-school booster because there is less risk of serious complications in older children. In addition, the change in 1990 was made in response to medical studies and surveys that showed that babies immunized at this younger age were less likely to have reactions to the vaccines, and could benefit from acquiring an adequate and immediate immune response.

In the UK, the schedule for childhood immunizations is:

2 months	diphtheria, tetanus, whooping cough (DTP)
	Haemophilus influenzae type B (Hib), polio
3 months	as above
4 months	as above
12–15 months	measles, mumps, rubella (MMR)
3–5 years	diphtheria, tetanus, polio (booster)
	measles, mumps, rubella (MMR booster)
Around 13 years	tuberculosis (BCG)
16/18 years	tetanus (booster)

In Australia, the schedule is the same as the UK for the first four months. At 12 months a child will receive the MMR vaccine and Hib booster, and at 18 months a DTP booster (and Hib booster if not received at 12 months). At school entry age children receive a DTP, polio and MMR booster. Hepatitis B immunization has been endorsed for all Australian infants but isn't yet part of the routine schedule. In the first year following the introduction of the Hib vaccine, the incidence of the disease in Australia was reduced by 94 per cent.

See page 114 for the recommended immunization schedule in the United States.

Administering the vaccine

All immunizations, with the exception of the polio vaccine which is usually given by mouth, are injected into the muscle, usually in the upper arm or the upper thigh in babies or children. Having an injection invariably makes a baby or young child cry for a moment or two. This is usually because of the surprise of the immediate pain, which is short lived, combined with the indignation that you, a parent, have somehow been the cause of it. Distressing though this is for a parent to witness, it is momentary, and for very young babies and older children alike, a cuddle is very reassuring. If, as a parent, you prefer not to witness the actual injection, tell the health visitor, nurse or doctor that you would prefer someone else to hold your child during the procedure, and comfort them yourself afterwards. Taking a friend with you can also be helpful.

Giving consent

In the UK you will be asked for your consent, verbal or written, for your baby or child to be immunized. You will probably be asked to sign your baby's or child's medical records, and the vaccine manufacturer's name, together with the lot and batch number, should also be entered on these records. If this isn't done routinely, ask for this information to be included. It may also be worthwhile making a note of it on your own family records. Consent is also necessary for older children, who may be offered immunization through a school health service, although if a parent or guardian has been informed of a forthcoming date when vaccination is being carried out, a child's presence at school that day may imply consent. The school may then request a written note stating that you do not wish your child to receive this vaccination if this is the case.

It is also considered legal for a child under the age of 16 to give consent provided he or she fully understands the benefits and risks involved. In the same way, a child in this position is also entitled to refuse immunization. It is difficult enough for an adult to fully understand both the benefits and risks of immunization, so where immunization is offered through a school, the parent or guardian of the child should be involved in the decision.

Reasons not to have your child immunized

Below are the clinical reasons why immunization may not be recommended for your child. They should be discussed with your health visitor, nurse or doctor and a decision made about whether or not it is appropriate for your child to be immunized:

* *Your baby or child has a high fever.*
* *There has been a previous bad reaction to immunization.*
* *Your child has had a severe allergic reaction to eggs.*
* *Your child is having, or has had, treatment for cancer.*
* *Your child has had any sort of fit or convulsion.*
* *You child has a bleeding disorder.*
* *Your child has had previous convulsions, or there is a family history of unstable neurological disorders, such as epilepsy.*
* *Your child, or a close family member, has any illness relating to the immune system, for example HIV or AIDS.*
* *Your child, or a close family member, is taking any immuno-suppressive drugs or a high dose of steroids, for any reason.*

It is likely that you have got to know your local family doctor, clinic nurse or health visitor over a period of time so that any longstanding health problems or worries are known to them and can be reviewed when decisions surrounding immunization need to be made. However, if you have just moved to a new area, or there has been a change in your family's medical care, you may have to check that all the information about your family, baby or child is available. It is always worthwhile talking through your concerns to be sure that you have provided all the information that might be relevant, and to help you make an informed choice about immunization for your child.

In an ideal world your doctor or health practitioner will be able to advise you and talk through your individual concerns about immunization for your baby. However, you may feel it necessary to gather your own information about immunization in order to make choices you are happy with. Ironically, you are likely to find more extensive information opposing immunization than advocating it. Support groups are seldom set up by parents who want to encourage other parents to immunize. In most cases those organizations claiming to offer impartial advice have been set up by individuals who have a personal reason to oppose immunization. Much of the material supplied by these groups is very emotive and it can be difficult not to feel vulnerable about your own baby's health when reading it. It is important when reviewing information about immunization to assess both sides, but it is also important to finally make your own decision, and feel happy about it. Then, on the basis of your decision, it becomes possible to assertively opt for, or reject, immunization for your child. And remember, routine childhood immunization is only recommended: you are under no legal obligation to immunize your child and can refuse, or you can opt to have your child immunized at an age other than that set out in the recommended schedule.

Premature babies

Premature babies have less protection than those born at full term, because the transfer of passive immunity (provided by antibodies in the mother's blood) occurs between weeks 28 and 40 of pregnancy. And even if antibodies to whooping cough were transferred from mother to baby, they appear to offer little or no protection from the disease. The time when immunization is given to protect premature babies should be calculated from the actual date of birth, not the expected date of delivery. For some babies this will mean they are immunized while still in the special care or neonatal baby unit.

Common reactions to immunization

Some children show no reaction at all to immunization, while some can seem quite unwell. It isn't always possible to predict accurately how babies or children will react, or what other illnesses or upsets immunization may coincide with. However, the first two symptoms listed below are experienced in about half of all immunized children, but these shouldn't last longer than a day or two:

* *a degree of tenderness and swelling at the site of the injection*
* *mild to moderate fever*
* *loss of appetite*
* *vomiting*
* *fussiness*
* *drowsiness*

If at any time during the first 48 hours following immunization the following symptoms occur, contact your doctor immediately:

* *high-pitched, persistent crying, for more than three hours*
* *unusual limpness, or paleness*
* *any convulsion*

* excessive sleepiness plus drowsiness and lack of alertness when awake
* rectal temperature of 40°C or 104°F

What to do if your child is unwell following immunization

Treat your baby or child as you would if they were showing symptoms of any illness. If there is a fever, cool your baby down by removing any excess clothing and sponging with tepid water if necessary. Give infant paracetamol in the recommended dose (or as advised by your doctor if your baby is under three months old) to both reduce a fever and provide pain relief for a sore injection site. The dose can be repeated after four to six hours, with no more than four doses in 24 hours. If you want to give a homeopathic remedy, consult a qualified homeopath for advice before immunization is given, so that you have the appropriate remedy for your child to hand (see Chapter 6).

TEPID SPONGING

To cool a baby down, tepid sponging can be very effective. In a draught-free room, remove your baby's clothes and lay him or her on a soft towel. Using tepid water – cool water makes the blood capillaries at the skin's surface contract, so keeping heat in – wring out a flannel, or squeeze a sponge in the water and gently stroke over your baby's limbs and body, the head and face, the back and neck, rinsing the cloth or sponge regularly. Wrap your child loosely in a dry towel, and check the temperature.

Repeat if necessary 30 minutes later, but don't allow your baby to cool too quickly.

Travelling abroad

It is not possible to stipulate exactly what should be considered when travelling abroad with children, because – as for adults – different countries have different requirements. The recommendation therefore is to ask your doctor for advice. Some specialist organizations may also be able to help. In the UK, for example, MASTA (Medical Advisory Service for Travellers Abroad), based at the London School of Hygiene and Tropical Medicine, run a Traveller's Health Line. (See Useful Addresses for details.)

Not all advice offered is for immunization. Often, if routine immunization for polio, tetanus, etc. is up to date, recommendations may only be made for passive immunity with gammaglobulin for hepatitis, for example, or occasionally some countries may require immunization for diseases such as yellow fever. But the precautions that are relevant for adults can be inappropriate for babies and children, so it is important to get specific advice.

3

Infectious diseases and immunization

Immunization can prevent, or minimize, the risk of catching a number of infectious diseases which were once commonplace in childhood. Infants and children are obviously most at risk from the infectious diseases so commonly associated with childhood, especially once they start school and spend extended periods of time in each other's company.

Prior to immunization, the only way to acquire immunity before adulthood was to get the disease. There was also the expectation that children would routinely get illnesses like mumps, chickenpox, measles and whooping cough. Children were nursed at home, or hospitalized, and families quarantined, until it was realized that the most infectious period of a disease was usually the period before symptoms appeared. This is why, if your child has even a relatively mild attack of chickenpox, for example, it is important to alert others who have been in close contact in the preceding couple of weeks. It is particularly important to alert pregnant mothers as chickenpox can cause quite serious problems in unborn babies, as can German measles (rubella), which is often difficult to diagnose because the rash may only be slight. German measles can cause congenital rubella syndrome, which may result in hearing, heart and brain damage in the unborn child if a pregnant mother catches it during the first three months of pregnancy.

Although the common childhood illnesses can make a child sick, and can be quite serious in babies under one, adults can suffer too, often more seriously. It was therefore thought advantageous for children to get these illnesses 'over and done with' in childhood, in order to acquire the immunity necessary to protect adult health. But this meant that for each illness a baby or child needed to be nursed at home for up to two weeks – something that is difficult to consider today for many modern families where both parents work.

On an individual basis, it is possible to reduce the risk of catching a disease through immunization, or it can be done collectively through relying on herd immunity, which in turn depends on a requisite percentage of the overall population being immunized. When immunization rates fall below a certain level, there is then the possibility of the disease becoming prevalent again. For example, in the UK during the years 1951–53, only 30 per cent of babies were immunized against diphtheria during their first year. This means that currently there is a gap in immunity levels among the adult population, with around one third or more of adults over the age of 35 being susceptible to infection, should it occur. Diphtheria is still endemic in many countries around the world, and all recent cases in the UK have come in from outside. Although the potential for a problem in the UK does exist, the situation is being closely monitored and there is as yet no cause for concern.

The following information outlines the main illnesses covered by the current childhood immunization schedule in the UK and numerous other countries worldwide (including the US and Australia), and what role immunization may play in protecting your child.

Meningitis

Meningitis describes an inflammation of the meninges, the membranes covering the brain and spinal cord, which can be caused by a number of micro-organisms, both bacterial and viral. Bacterial meningitis is more life threatening than viral meningitis, but can be treated by antibiotics if diagnosed in time. The most common cause of bacterial meningitis today, since the introduction of routine immunization against the Hib bacterium (see below), is meningococcal meningitis. Viral meningitis tends to occur in cyclical fashion and in local outbreaks, usually during the winter months.

Following recent media campaigns in the UK, most parents of young children are familiar with the symptoms of meningitis – abnormal drowsiness, fever, over-sensitivity to light, vomiting, increased crying – but the illness still raises concern because in the early stages it can be difficult to say what might be the cause of these symptoms. However, babies, children and even adults can get seriously ill very fast and as recovery is often dependent on prompt treatment, this is very worrying. The appearance of a meningitis rash, flat pink or purple spots that don't fade when a drinking glass is pressed against them, indicates blood poisoning, which can be fatal without prompt treatment.

Short-term protection against one strain of meningococcal meningitis can be provided by immunization during local outbreaks, but the Hib vaccine is offered routinely and offers protection against *Haemophilus influenzae* type B, a bacterium that can cause meningitis, epiglottitis (a potentially fatal form of croup that can obstruct the airway), septicaemia (blood poisoning), pericarditis (inflammation of the membrane which covers the heart) and otitis media (infection of the middle ear). When Hib was first discovered in 1892, it was thought to be the cause of influenza (which is where Hib originally took its name) but this was later found to be untrue.

Between 1 and 5 per cent of the population in the UK are thought to be carriers of Hib, the rate being highest in children under five years old. Through this exposure most people become immune to Hib during the first few years of life. Babies are born with a degree of passive immunity to Hib, with antibodies being passed from the mother after around 32 weeks of pregnancy. Babies may also be protected to a lesser extent by breastfeeding. However, from the age of about three months this protective effect begins to decline.

Before the vaccination was introduced in the UK in 1993, there were around 1,600 Hib infections each year, with 60 deaths. By the age of five, 1 in 600 children had had the disease, and 1 in 800 children developed meningitis. One study which followed a group of children up to the age of five who had had the Hib infection found that 4 per cent of the children had died during the acute stage of the illness and 8 per cent had significant after-effects including hearing loss, learning difficulties and cerebral palsy. In the United States, vaccination has been routine since 1990. There had been around 20,000 cases of Hib-related disease annually; this declined until in 1998 there were 125 reported cases.

Vaccination

Babies in the UK are first given the Hib vaccine at two months, and then again at three and four months, and at 12 months in the US.

Measles

This is one of the most infectious of the viral illnesses, and it was very common in childhood prior to its inclusion in the vaccination programme. If children without immunity come into contact with measles they are more than likely to catch it, however good their general health is. The incubation period is 10 to 14 days, after which symptoms include fever, runny nose, dry cough and red watering eyes. The rash of flat blotchy red patches appears about three to four days later, first of all on the face and behind the ears and then spreading to cover the whole body. Tiny white spots with a red base, Koplik's spots, can sometimes be seen inside the cheeks a couple of days prior to the external rash appearing. Your child is infectious before the rash appears, and for about five days afterwards, so although staying away from susceptible people is important, for family members it's probably too late.

I had had measles as a child, and was still breastfeeding my eight-month-old daughter when she caught measles. I couldn't believe it, and never did work out where she caught it from. She was quite poorly with it, and off her food for a long time, but didn't suffer any complications. Apart from the rash, it was like a really bad cold and cough, but I'd rather she hadn't caught it at all as I was pretty worried when the doctor diagnosed measles. Luckily my son, aged four, didn't catch it so I'm grateful that his immunization worked.
Alison, mother to Josh, 4, and Rose, 11 months

Many children who get measles recover well, but for a significant few there are complications including otitis media (infection of the middle ear) and bacterial pneumonia, which can be treated with antibiotics, and in about 1 in 1,000 cases encephalitis occurs. This inflammation of the brain, caused either by a spread of the measles virus to the brain or an abnormal immune response, can cause long-term damage, although for most children the outcome will depend on the severity of symptoms and whether or not any permanent brain damage has occurred.

Although in a previously healthy, well-nourished child measles is not likely to be a serious illness, there are numerous children within any population who do not fall into this category. The risk of developing complications also increases in children whose health is already compromised in some way. However, between the years 1970 and 1983 in the UK, half the deaths from measles did occur in previously healthy children, of whom 90 per cent were of an age at which they would have been offered immunization.

One rare complication of measles infection is that of SSPE (subacute sclerosing panencephalitis), which causes inflammation and destruction of the nervous system, and death. The measles virus can lie dormant and be reactivated up to seven years later, causing SSPE. Between the years 1970 and 1989 in England and Wales, SSPE occurred at a rate of 4 per 100,000 cases of measles. The risk of this complication is 18 times higher in children who catch measles before the age of one than in those who have measles after the age of five. The risk of SSPE occurring after vaccination against measles was found to be 29 times lower than the risk following a natural attack.

Vaccination

The measles vaccine is offered routinely at around 12 months in the US and 13 months in the UK, in combination with that for mumps and rubella, as the MMR vaccine. It is not given before the first year because any remaining maternal antibodies, providing passive immunity, can interfere with antibody production stimulated by the vaccine. An MMR booster is offered between the ages of four and six, and three and five, respectively.

SIDE EFFECTS AND COMPLICATIONS

The MMR vaccine, like all medicines, is constantly monitored for safety and effectiveness. It has, however, been the subject of extensive debate and concern because of a possible link with both childhood autism and Crohn's disease. The dangers of the MMR vaccine causing encephalitis were found to be at a rate of 1 in 1 million doses, which is similar to the rate of encephalitis occurring for no known reason in the same age group.

The possible link between measles and Crohn's disease, and the MMR vaccine and Crohn's disease, was raised in 1995 when research carried out by a group of doctors in the UK was published. This research compared the incidence of Crohn's disease in a group of people who had received the measles vaccine in 1964 with the incidence in two other groups. While the researchers found an association, they also stated that 'it does not show a causal relation'.

Two studies published later, in 1997, in contrast showed no link. And another study showed no link between measles infection before birth and Crohn's disease. The World Health Organization, in reviewing all the current scientific evidence, can find no proof of a causal link between the two. Research also continues to try and establish whether there is any link between the measles virus and inflammatory bowel disease, but so far this doesn't appear to be the case.

We went to live in the States, because of my husband's posting, for two years when our children were four and five. Because there's a family history of Crohn's disease, and because there was some concern about the MMR vaccination and a link to this, we had been advised in the UK not to give it at that time. However, in spite of our medical documentation from the UK, the school authorities where we were living were adamant: our children couldn't attend school without having been immunized against measles. As far as they were concerned, there was insufficient medical evidence to prevent immunization. If we had had religious grounds for not immunizing, we would have been fine – but the medical reasons were not sufficient. It was quite a dilemma, and in the end we had them immunized, having checked out lots of other available data, but it was very tricky.

Maria, mother to Christopher, 6, and Michael, 5

Mumps

Generally considered to be a mild viral illness, with an incubation period of 14 to 24 days, mumps causes fever and the characteristic swelling of the parotid salivary glands in the neck. This can be very sore and lasts for four to eight days. Swelling of the testes can sometimes occur but, contrary to popular belief, this rarely leads to infertility even in older boys and men.

Mumps can occasionally give rise to meningitis and encephalitis, so if your child complains of a continuous severe headache your doctor may want to suggest a lumbar puncture to rule out these conditions. Mumps used to be the commonest cause of viral meningitis, affecting around 1 in 400 children. In most cases rest at home will help a sick child, with regular doses of infant paracetamol if necessary to reduce fever and pain, and lots of fluids – although avoid fruit or citrus juices that stimulate saliva and cause pain from the glands.

Vaccination

The mumps vaccine was introduced in 1988, combined with the measles and rubella injection. Before then, mumps epidemics occurred every three years in the UK. In the UK and US the vaccine is given to babies at 12 to 15 months, as part of the MMR vaccine, with a booster between the ages of three and five.

SIDE EFFECTS AND COMPLICATIONS

Initially there was some concern that the vaccine was linked to a risk of aseptic (viral) meningitis and extensive research was carried out: all paediatricians were asked to report on hospitalized cases of meningoencephalitis occurring in children under 16 within six weeks of receiving the MMR vaccine. The overall risk was found to be 4 in 1 million children but in a number of specific areas it was much higher, and in one area it was as high as 1 in 4,000. Further research found that this was linked to the use of a vaccine containing the Urabe strain of the virus, and since this was dropped from use, no further case of meningitis has been found to be linked to the mumps vaccine.

Rubella

This is an innocuous viral disease that often passes without notice. There may be a slight fever, and a rash of small, flat pink spots that can start behind the ears but tend to merge into a flushed appearance lasting around three days before fading. Unlike scarlet fever, the rash doesn't fade when pressed. With no other real symptoms, this illness can be virtually over before parents realize their child has been infected. A doctor will look for tender, swollen glands at the back of the neck at the base of the skull, and may send a blood sample to a laboratory to check the diagnosis. Very rarely is there a link to encephalitis or to thrombocytopenia, where the platelets (clotting agents) in the blood fall abnormally low and bleeding into the skin and prolonged bleeding after injury may occur.

Rubella is included in the immunization programme because of the very serious risk to an unborn baby if its mother catches rubella in the first few months of pregnancy. The link was discovered in 1941 by an Australian eye doctor called Gregg, who made the connection between a surprisingly large number of infants with cataracts and the rubella caught by their mothers in Australia's 1940 epidemic. It was also found to be the case in Sweden, the US and the UK, and the link between rubella and congenital cataracts was made. Then the link between congenital deafness and heart disease was noted, and a definition of congenital rubella syndrome was established. In the US in 1964–5 a major rubella outbreak resulted in around 20,000 babies born who were rubella damaged, and the need for prevention of this seemingly innocent disease was highlighted.

In 1982 research published showed that women who caught rubella in the first 12 weeks of pregnancy had an 80 per cent chance of the baby being born with congenital rubella syndrome. At 13–14 weeks of pregnancy the risk dropped to 67 per cent, and steadily declined until the risk was 25 per cent at 26 weeks of pregnancy. The most common problems associated with congenital rubella are deafness, heart defects, cataracts and other sight problems, learning difficulties and cerebral palsy.

Vaccination

The vaccine was introduced in the UK in 1970, initially for school girls and susceptible older women, and the National Congenital Rubella Surveillance Programme was set up in 1971 to monitor its safety and effectiveness. It is now given as part of the MMR vaccine at 12–15 months, with a booster between the ages of three and five, or four and six in the US.

One dose of the vaccine gives permanent protection in 95 per cent of cases, but there have been reports of people who were previously immune (either through vaccination or having had the disease) and have lost that immunity. So it is still a good idea for women planning pregnancy to check out their immune status, which can be done by a simple blood test. Rubella vaccination should not be given to pregnant women, or given less than one month before getting pregnant because of the possible risk of damage.

SIDE EFFECTS AND COMPLICATIONS

Any reaction to the vaccine is usually mild and temporary, occurring between one and three weeks later. At one time there was thought to be a link between the vaccine and an increase in arthritis, but several recent studies have not confirmed this. And while one research study in 1995 suggested that the risk of thrombocytopenia after vaccination was 1 in 29,000, this was a risk eight times lower than that attached to the actual illness.

Polio (poliomyelitis)

There's seldom any information about polio nowadays in childcare books, except as a footnote to information about immunization, because it is no longer considered to be a disease that children are likely to get. Polio is, however, a viral infection of the intestines that can affect the central nervous system, resulting in paralysis in a small number of cases.

Polio has an incubation period of around seven to 14 days, and the early symptoms are mild – fever and headache – and improve after a few days. This may be the disease's only effect, but in some cases about a week later symptoms recur with neck stiffness and other signs of meningeal irritation. Widespread muscle paralysis can follow, including paralysis of the diaphragm which stops breathing and kills unless artificial respiration aids are used, which gave rise to the horror stories in the 1940s and '50s about 'iron lungs'. Nerve cells in the lumbar region of the spinal cord are most commonly affected, and still today you see people in their fifties walking with a limp as a consequence of childhood polio. Recovery is gradual, and requires total bed rest for a long period of time, followed by physiotherapy. In some cases paralysis continues and a limb remains useless for life.

The number of polio cases in the UK from the 1920s to the 1990s indicates regular incidence with occasional peaks until the late 1940s, when the incidence soared from less than 2,000 notifications a year to almost 8,000, and from then on it remained high until the routine introduction of the vaccine in the late 1950s. The rate of incidence then fell dramatically until polio was almost eradicated in the UK by the late 1960s. It's easy to forget now, with only memories of what a devastating disease it was, that polio was a cause of great dread among parents in the 1950s in the UK, and elsewhere. In the US there were 16,316 cases and 1,879 deaths between the years 1957 and 1964; the vaccine was introduced in 1955. Infant paralysis, as polio was also known, was a great terror to previous generations.

Vaccination

In the UK, polio vaccination is received as a live oral polio vaccine, whereas in France, Finland, the Netherlands and

Scandinavia a dead oral polio vaccine is used. In the US, Israel and Denmark, however, the dead oral polio vaccine is used in combination with the live one. The UK continues to use the live vaccine because it gives wider immunity, behaving in a way more similar to the actual disease. The dead, or inactivated, polio virus may not be so efficient at preventing intestinal infections. So in each country there are important considerations about which vaccine to use.

In the UK babies are vaccinated at two, three and four months, with a booster between the ages of three and five. In the US vaccinations are at two, four, and six to 18 months, with a booster between four and six years of age.

SIDE EFFECTS AND COMPLICATIONS

Concern has also been expressed about the use in the UK of a live oral vaccine, which results in the virus being excreted in a baby's stools for up to six weeks after vaccination. While the majority of people are immune, there may be family members and others who aren't, so it's important to take extra care with disposing of nappy contents and washing hands after changing nappies. Taking recently vaccinated babies swimming, where accidents might occur in the water, poses no threat to others because of the dilution in such a large quantity of chlorinated water.

Diphtheria

This disease sounds like something out of a Victorian novel, and is rarely seen nowadays in developed countries although it is still endemic among much of the world's population. It is caused by a highly infectious bacterium, and is spread by water droplets. The incubation period is two to four days, and the first symptoms are a slightly raised temperature and a sore throat, with some swelling of the lymph nodes in the neck. What then happens is a membrane forms over the back of the throat which obstructs breathing and produces a powerful toxin that damages the tissues of the heart and nerves. In severe cases and without prompt antibiotic treatment, many patients die.

Although the incidence of diphtheria declined in the UK from 1915 onwards, thanks to improved sanitation in particular, there were still 41,042 cases recorded in 1942, when immunization was introduced, with 1,827 deaths. By 1946, when 60 per cent of children had been vaccinated, the number of deaths had fallen to 472. Nowadays, in all recorded cases in the UK the disease has come in from abroad: in 1994, for example, a 14-year-old boy who had recently returned to the UK from Pakistan died of diphtheria. However, it is still a serious problem in many countries; for example, in the new, independent states of the former Soviet Union in 1994 an epidemic resulted in 47,802 cases and 1,746 deaths.

Vaccination

Babies are normally given the vaccine as part of the DTP vaccine at two, three and four months in the UK and two, four and six months in the US, with a booster between the ages of three and five, and four and six.

SIDE EFFECTS AND COMPLICATIONS

See general information on page 22.

Tetanus

The tetanus bug is found in soil and dust, particularly where there is also animal manure. Infection usually follows a deep puncture wound, or a gun shot wound, or where there is a foreign body that needs removal. This provides a good site for the bacterium *Clostridium tetani* to breed. The bug reproduces anaerobically, i.e. when there is no oxygen present, so contamination begins after the wound has begun to heal. The resulting toxins can cause extreme muscle contractions, which give rise to the old-fashioned name for tetanus, 'lock jaw', because in very bad cases the muscle contractions caused an obstruction to breathing, and consequently death. Being healthy and fit offers no protection against this particular illness, and anyone who is unimmunized is at risk.

Vaccination

Immunization against tetanus is routinely given as part of the 'triple vaccine' (DTP) against diphtheria, whooping cough and tetanus.

Tetanus immunization was routine in the UK among the armed forces from 1938, but began among children from 1961. Now in the UK, the group at greatest risk because of non-immunization are women in their fifties, unless they have been vaccinated as adults.

Even if your child has been immunized, if there is a deep, dirty wound it is always best to see your doctor or go to an accident and emergency department for treatment. It may be necessary to give a booster injection to be sure. Although a course of immunization is given in infancy, boosters are usually given before school entry and leaving school, and are recommended every 10 years throughout adult life. Many people don't get round to having routine boosters, however, so they are usually recommended if a deep wound has occurred.

SIDE EFFECTS AND COMPLICATIONS
See general information on page 22.

Whooping cough

Also called pertussis (consequently the 'P' in the DTP vaccination – diphtheria, tetanus and pertussis), this is a bacterial disease that is now uncommon in developed countries with childhood immunization programmes. Although anyone of any age can get it, 90 per cent of cases in the UK tend to occur in unimmunized children under the age of five, and it is most common during winter months.

The incubation period is around seven days, and symptoms of whooping cough tend to occur in two stages. During the first stage there is typically a slight fever, runny nose and a short, dry cough which can be worse at night. This can last for about 7 to 10 days, after which bouts of extended coughing occur, during both the day and night. At the end of each bout there is often a sharp breathing in, which can cause the characteristic 'whooping' noise that gives the illness its name, although whooping often doesn't occur in babies. Vomiting can often occur after bouts of coughing, too. This second stage can last anything up to 8 to 12 weeks.

41

The severity of the illness varies. It can be very mild, but when it's bad it isn't pleasant, and can be dangerous in very young babies. A bad bout of whooping cough can also be very debilitating, particularly because the endless night-time coughing disturbs sleep. This tends to be the main problem for older children, whose health over a long period of time can be quite badly affected. During a bad bout of the illness, a child will require a lot of nursing, rest and support. Very young babies really don't manage the illness well, unless it's very mild. Antibiotics can help, but only if given early enough during the course of the illness. Coughing can continue for several months, and can recur following a subsequent viral upper respiratory chest infection, although permanent lung damage is rare.

Vaccination

Vaccination against whooping cough was introduced in the UK in the 1940s and is now part of the DTP vaccine given to babies. A later booster is now thought unnecessary in the UK; in the US it is recommended at four to six years. A full course is reckoned to protect against the disease in 80 per cent of cases, and for those who do catch it, the illness is likely to be less severe.

SIDE EFFECTS AND COMPLICATIONS

The whooping cough vaccine has generated much controversy. In 1974, a paper was published by doctors at the Great Ormond Street Hospital for Sick Children in London, which suggested that there was a link between the vaccination and epilepsy and learning disorders. Following this there was, quite understandably, a dramatic fall in the uptake of immunization and a corresponding increase of 100,000 extra cases of the illness between 1977 and 1980.

In response to this concern in the UK, a major study was set up called the National Childhood Encephalopathy Study. Over a three-year period, this looked at children between the ages of two months and three years who had been hospitalized with a serious, acute illness of the nervous system. For every child who fell into this category and was studied, two other children were studied as a control. All sorts of other information was studied as well as immunization histories, and the results were published in 1981. These concluded that the risk of an acute illness of the nervous system, i.e. encephalitis, was 1 in 110,000 immunizations, and the risk of permanent brain damage was 1 in 310,000. These figures are in sharp contrast to those of children who have whooping cough, where the link to brain disease is 1 in 10,000 cases.

And the studies have continued in both the UK and the US. One of the largest reviews of all the literature covering the adverse effects of both the whooping cough and rubella vaccinations was carried out in the States by the Institute of Medicine. This wide-ranging review took over two years, looking at published and unpublished material, case studies, case reports, epidemiological studies, and laboratory research. The final conclusion was that there was insufficient evidence to indicate that the DTP vaccine was a definite cause of a variety of problems including aseptic meningitis, attention deficit disorder, long-term damage to the nervous system, juvenile diabetes, learning difficulties, haemolytic anaemia, and others.

In the UK, in 1993, when Kenneth Best was awarded damages of £2.75 million from a vaccine manufacturer, it was because he had received his vaccination from a specific batch that had failed its safety test. The judgement was awarded on the basis that he shouldn't have received whooping cough vaccine from a damaged batch, and that this particular batch should never have been released for use.

In view of the concerns raised about the whooping cough vaccine, since 1974 seven major committees have analysed and re-analysed the risks to the nervous system. There has been no evidence to confirm that the vaccine causes brain damage.

Tuberculosis (TB)

Although TB is strongly associated with poverty and malnutrition, and has been in strong decline in the UK and other developed nations, there has been a new risk with the rise of immigrant populations. As with many diseases, TB can be most damaging in childhood. Although it can be a relatively minor respiratory disease, and can be indistinguishable from other diseases, it can affect the lungs. In some cases TB can spread to other areas of the body – the kidneys, spinal cord and brain, and the bones. It is treatable with a potent combination of antibiotics, not themselves without some adverse effects.

Vaccination

The BCG (Bacillus Calmette-Guérin) vaccine was introduced in the 1950s, and was for a long time given to school children in the UK at around the age of 14. This was because a Medical

Research Council trial, which began in 1950, indicated that this was very effective at preventing TB for at least 15 years. Currently in the UK it has been suggested that there is no longer any need to vaccinate routinely, as this is no longer cost effective. And in spite of guidelines from the UK's Department of Health, policies on BCG vaccination vary among the different local health authorities around the country.

Another problem with TB vaccination programmes is that reports of the vaccine's ability to provide protection vary so widely – being anything from 0 to 80 per cent effective. These figures resulted from ten trials carried out throughout the world, although there is no real agreement about why they should be so variable. However, one trial in North America carried out to assess the effectiveness of the vaccine when given to newborn babies estimated it to be between 75 and 80 per cent effective.

SIDE EFFECTS AND COMPLICATIONS

Immunization with the BCG vaccine invariably leaves a small scar at the site of injection, so this is often placed in the flesh under the arm rather than at the shoulder. A small pimple usually forms after about two weeks, increases in size, then crusts over to eventually form a white scar. Anything more severe than this is probably the result of a faulty injection technique, where the vaccine was given too deeply.

Hepatitis B

Although part of the routine childhood immunization programme in the US, it is not in the UK; however, it is becomingly increasingly common in the UK to screen pregnant mothers for the hepatitis B virus. It can be present in body fluids – blood, saliva, semen, vaginal secretions, and breastmilk – so a baby born to an infected mother would be at high risk. While the UK is still considered a country of low incidence, in some areas antenatal clinics have picked up 1 per cent of mothers carrying the virus.

Hepatitis is a serious disease that can cause chronic liver damage and death. It is also considered to be second only to tobacco as a risk associated with cancer. There are an estimated 400–500 million hepatitis B carriers in the world today, so it is a growing problem and is the reason why there is constant monitoring and debate about the inclusion of hepatitis B vaccine in a childhood immunization programme.

Vaccination

In the UK vaccination is recommended to babies of infected mothers at birth, then again at 18 months of age. In the US, universal immunization of all infants at birth has been recommended, while in Italy immunization is recommended at birth and during early adolescence.

SIDE EFFECTS AND COMPLICATIONS

Any side effects will tend to be mild. There may be some soreness or redness at the site of the injection. See also general information on page 22.

4

Boost your child's immune system – Nutrition

Nutrition

All parents, quite naturally, want to give their child the best start in life. This may have begun consciously before birth, with the mother-to-be taking supplements of folic acid and eating a diet rich in protein and fatty acids, keeping fit and consciously relaxing. It may be that by trying to create a harmonious, stress-free pregnancy, and by trying to reduce the traumatic impact of labour and birth on the baby, the chance of a good physical and emotional start to life is enhanced. But this is only the beginning of the long journey parents and their growing children make together, during which time there is a great deal that can be done to promote and enhance positive health and build a well-functioning immune system that will be of lasting benefit throughout life.

Although initially dependent on adult care, babies are born with fantastic survival mechanisms, many of which are instinctive. For example, the ability to cry when hungry or in discomfort alerts caring adults to their needs. And the quickly-learnt ability to smile in response to another creates a two-way attachment between infant and caregiver. Some survival mechanisms, however, such as the immune system, which is activated in part by exposure to the outside world are physical. During the first year of life, and the early development of the immune system, there is a great deal that can be done to support its development naturally. It is worth thinking about how you can enhance these options and ensure that the choices you make as a parent help rather than hinder this process. Some of this is related to the diet and food choices we provide our children, which will influence them in the way they eat and enjoy food, probably for the rest of their lives.

Much of what is outlined below will be familiar to any parent, but the focus is on developing immunity in particular and understanding the specific contribution that diet makes to its development. Early parenthood can leave many parents feeling vulnerable and insecure as they try to make decisions, knowing that some could have repercussions on their child's health in later life. As with anything, we can only make choices based on what we know and what we believe is relevant to us and our children at that time.

Recent food scares surrounding BSE, salmonella, genetically modified foods, and the use of organophosphates in the food chain, for example, can make the process of food selection a nerve-wracking process. Children's nutritional needs are different to those of an adult, so it is important to be properly informed if you wish to make specific dietary changes that you feel may be to the long-term benefit of your child. For example, if you want your baby to follow a vegetarian diet but are not sure about what is acceptable in terms of nutrition, then ask for a referral to a paediatric dietician, who can advise you.

Given what we know about our own health or that of our immediate family, we may have some idea of the genetic predisposition of our child. For example, although the susceptibility to allergies appears to be increasing, it is unlikely that your child will have a true food allergy if there is no family history of allergy.

Breastfeeding

The general message from childcare experts is that 'breast is best' for babies, but it isn't always clear why, or for how long, or what exactly is gained by breastfeeding exclusively for the first four to six months of life.

The society in which we live has a very mixed attitude towards breastfeeding, and as a consequence it is unusual to see women breastfeeding their babies in public. The message many women receive is that breastfeeding is frowned upon, that it is difficult, and that it must be done to the exclusion of any other type of feeding, and therefore it will restrict them considerably. The truth is that breastfeeding is convenient and natural. It can be done at any time, requires no complicated sterilization routines, and once established can offer a flexible and discreet way to feed your baby for the first few months, and for longer if wanted. You can breastfeed exclusively or, after feeding is established, you can mix breast with bottlefeeding for greater flexibility, using either expressed breastmilk or infant formula. Then, after solids are introduced at around four months, you can mix and match however you like. Even after the introduction of solids, breastfeeding can continue and, even at this reduced intake, it will continue to contribute positively to an infant's health.

In terms of promoting health and boosting immunity in new babies, there's nothing to beat human breastmilk. It is the most suitable first food for babies as it contains all the nutrients needed for healthy growth, in the right proportions, and is readily available without the worry of sterilizing equipment. Infant milk formulas made from modified cow's milk are a close substitute for human breastmilk but in order to emulate it contain lots of additional ingredients. Even so, they cannot contain the hidden health advantages of breastmilk, from which babies benefit greatly.

Even though I had to go back to work at six weeks, I was very clear that I wanted to breastfeed Gemma. She was breastfed exclusively at first, then when I went back to work she had bottles of formula but I still fed her myself morning and night. Now she's weaned onto solids, and drinking from a cup – but I still feed her myself first thing in the morning and to settle her at night. No one told me this would be possible, but I'm really glad I persevered even when it was quite tricky when I first had to leave her: I still produced masses of milk during the day for the first few days and it was pretty uncomfortable – but it's been great. Now she's almost a year old, and seems very healthy.

Suzy, mother to Gemma, 11 months

What is unique about breastmilk is that it changes in response to a baby's needs, regulating the carbohydrate and fat content to meet the changing nutritional needs of a growing infant. The first milk, colostrum, which is produced during the first few days, is high in proteins and minerals but also includes the maternal antibodies that are crucial in providing passive immunity. This can help protect vulnerable newborns from illness until they have a chance to produce their own antibodies.

Because breastmilk contains not just antibodies but also anti-infective and antiviral properties, breastfed babies show greater resistance to tummy upsets, chest infections, ear infections and urine infections. Recent research has also shown that breastfed babies benefit from the continual antibody response their mothers have to prevailing infections. For example, in an environment of constant coughs and colds – especially during the winter when there are numerous respiratory tract viruses about – the baby benefits from and is protected in part by the mother's continual ability to produce her own antibodies and pass these on to her baby in her breastmilk. The immunoglobulins produced by the mother are extremely effective in all sorts of beneficial ways, including helping the gut to mature. This, in turn, has been shown to help prevent neonatal necrotizing enterocolitis, a serious but rare problem in the gut which can lead to perforation of the bowel. It is more common in preterm babies.

Also present in human breastmilk are the long-chain polyunsaturated fatty acids DHA (docosahexaenoic acid) and AA (arachidonic acid), which are essential to the healthy development of the brain, nervous tissue and the retina of the eye. Breastmilk is therefore particularly important for premature babies who aren't yet able to manufacture either DHA or AA from other essential fatty acids, linoleic acid and alpha-linoleic acid. Although some infant milk formula manufacturers have added DHA and AA to their product, the best way to ensure your baby gets these long-chain polyunsaturated fatty acids is to breastfeed. Research has also shown that babies who receive DHA and AA show higher cognitive intelligence at 10 months, measured against a control group. One study reported in the *Lancet* showed that the IQ of breastfed babies was generally eight points higher.

Another benefit of breastfeeding is that it helps in the 'switching on' of a baby's immune system. Research done in Italy suggests that long-term breastfeeding can actually help reduce the risk of developing multiple sclerosis. It has also been shown that babies who have been exclusively breastfed produce more antibodies in response to vaccination. In some way their immune system seems to be more responsive, and more mature in its response. Even though high levels of antibody production are no final guarantee of good health, they are an effective indicator of immune response, which contributes so greatly to an individual's ability to fight disease.

I'm not sure that my children really got fewer coughs and colds than other children, but it was very easy to comfort them when they were babies because I was breastfeeding. I do think that they seemed to recover quite quickly, and didn't seem to have the endless runny noses that some other babies seemed to suffer.

Claire, mother to Rose, 4, and Alex, 18 months

When it comes to the development of a strong and responsive immune system, it is significant that breastmilk contains high concentrations of vitamins A, C and E. Vitamin A is sometimes referred to as the growth vitamin, because it is essential for the production of growth hormone. In turn, growth hormone is essential for the activity of the thymus gland and for the production of T lymphocytes, a vital part of the immune system. Vitamin A is also important for keeping cell walls strong and thus more resistant to viral attack, particular in vulnerable areas like the gut and the genito-urinary and respiratory tracts. It is also necessary for the production of lysozyme, an antibacterial substance found in tears and other body secretions.

Vitamin C has effective antiviral properties, and also boosts prostaglandin production necessary for T-cell production. It detoxifies some bugs, reducing their impact, and has antibacterial properties, too. Vitamin E has an important role to play in boosting immunity, especially as it is needed for a normal antibody response. Like vitamin C, vitamin E also has antioxidant properties that help protect against air pollutants like car exhaust.

There may be fewer minerals present in human breastmilk than in its infant formula counterpart, but they are of a type that are more readily digested. This is particularly the case with iron and calcium. Babies are born with an iron reserve of about six months, but human breastmilk also contains lacto-ferrin, a protein that binds with the iron in breastmilk and makes it more easily accessible to your baby. Lacto-ferrin is also an effective anti-infective agent, so it has a dual purpose. Iron boosts overall resistance to infection, and vitamin C enhances its absorption, so again breastmilk is produced to work to the best advantage of your baby!

The increasing incidence of iron-deficiency anaemia amongst toddlers is a recent phenomenon. This has been blamed on many things: late weaning, the trends towards a vegetarian diet, no-beef diets because of BSE scares, infants being given tea as a drink (tea dramatically reduces the absorption of available dietary iron), etc. One of the symptoms of iron-deficiency anaemia, along with paleness, lethargy and vulnerability to infection is a distinct lack of appetite. This creates a vicious spiral, as it is hard to persuade a child who doesn't feel hungry to eat. A fussy eater who appears to dislike nearly all food may have a degree of iron-deficiency anaemia. If you suspect this, then it's worth consulting your doctor or health visitor. A simple blood test can confirm haemoglobin levels, and paediatric iron supplements are available. Don't, however, be tempted to give an iron supplement without professional advice as an excess of iron can be detrimental.

It never occured to me that Tom could be anaemic. He's always been a bit fussy about food, but it was only after a really bad winter, when he had a succession of colds, that he never seemed to be hungry. He seemed run down and too tired to enjoy life. Which was very much at odds with his previous boisterous character! The health visitor suggested a paediatric iron supplement, and within a couple of weeks he was a different child – and the most significant thing was that he developed a huge appetite in comparison to before!

Elaine, mother to Tom, 3

Calcium, too, is vital, and not just to build healthy bones and teeth. It enables the phagocytic cells produced by the body to attach themselves to foreign cells, in order to engulf and destroy them. Calcium is also important for the production of the necessary enzymes that make cytotoxic T-cells lethal to invaders. A mild fever in a baby, which enhances the positive role of macrophages in the blood to combat infection, requires calcium. Calcium also needs magnesium to be available to work, and these two minerals need to be in balance for each to be effective. Magnesium is essential for the production of antibodies, and a deficiency can create an increase in histamine levels and, as a consequence, allergic reactions.

Suffice to say that a breastfeeding baby gains an awful lot more than just nutrition from its food. And because a breastfeeding mother's body will disregard its own needs to ensure her baby receives the best, it is essential that she eats a balanced and nutritious diet — for her own health and wellbeing as well as that of her baby.

Diet

The positive link between breastfeeding and developing immunity can lead to anxiety about weaning, and a fear that it won't be possible ever again to provide your baby with such complete, adequate and safe food. Rest assured that, having given your baby the best start, this very good beginning can be built on positively as you start introducing solid foods.

Introducing your baby to solid foods means introducing him or her to one of the great pleasures of life, and being able to enjoy food is an important aspect of feeding. A great deal of our socializing is around food, and it offers an opportunity for families — in whatever shape or form — to enjoy spending time together. However, anxiety about feeding infants and children can all too often turn mealtimes into a battleground, so perhaps the key words are flexibility, diversity and knowledge. Flexibility in approach, diversity of foodstuffs offered, and knowledge about how to use food to help promote positive health in your child.

Learning to chew and swallow after merely sucking and swallowing is a new skill and takes time to learn, but it also gives you the chance to introduce your baby, slowly but surely, to food habits that will last a lifetime. Ultimately you want your baby to eat the same food as the rest of the family, so if your own dietary habits need reviewing – perhaps because you aren't eating enough fruit and vegetables – then this can be a beneficial opportunity for all the family.

Weaning, the period during which a gradual switch is made from a milk-only diet to solid foods, is the process of expanding the diet to include foods and drinks other than breastmilk or infant formula. In order to meet their nutritional needs, the majority of infants need nothing other than breastmilk or infant formula for the first four to six months of life. However, after this it's necessary to begin the introduction of more solid foods, allowing time for an infant to adapt to new tastes and textures. Chewing and swallowing are not necessary just in order to eat; this activity also encourages good dentition and strengthens the muscles of the face in preparation for speech. Breastfeeding can continue during and after weaning as long as the amount of breastmilk is reduced as the introduction of other foods increases. Babies who fill up on milk because it's a surefire way to get that lovely, full feeling may be disinclined to eat solids, but it's important to move towards a mixed, more 'calorie-dense' (high-calorie) diet of foods because after a while a baby would be unable to drink enough milk to get the calories for healthy growth.

In infancy, your child will need appropriate foods to support healthy growth. A low-fat, high-fibre diet, as recommended for adults, isn't suitable for children. Children need calorie-dense foods because they eat smaller quantities and, because they are growing rapidly, their energy needs are greater than ours. Full-fat products − milk, cheese, yoghurts − provide more calories, weight for weight, than low-fat products so are an example of calorie-dense foods. If there is an adequate source of fresh fruit and vegetables, cereals and pasta, then a source of fibre is already there and your child won't need any extra. Too much fibre in a child's diet encourages too swift a movement of food through the gut so there is insufficient time for all the nutrients to be absorbed.

Small children seldom eat large quantities of food and are unlikely to consume all they need from three main meals a day. They tend to 'graze' and may need snacks so that their overall daily intake is adequate. Some children may eat only a little one day, and more the next, so taking a weekly overview can sometimes be useful in assessing whether the quantity of what they are eating is adequate. If children seem fit and healthy, with plenty of energy, this will also be an indicator that their nutritional intake is adequate.

In order to provide a child with a healthy diet, it is necessary to offer a balance of foods. The Department of Health in the UK recommends that 50 per cent of energy needs should be provided by carbohydrates, 35 per cent by fats, and 15 per cent by protein. This gives you an idea of the proportions of foods needed, but how this actually equates to a possible daily intake of different foods is outlined below.

Starchy foods (carbohydrates) – bread, potatoes, pasta, rice, cereals: five to six servings (or portions or helpings)
Fruit and vegetables: four to five servings
Protein – red meat, poultry, fish, eggs, pulses, nuts: two to three servings
Dairy products – milk, yoghurt, cheese, fromage frais: two to three servings

Bear in mind that many foods contain a combination of components: for example, cheese contains fat and protein, and baked beans (opt for low-sugar varieties) contain starch and protein, so within this framework always go for diversity in what you offer. You can then feel confident that, in general, you are getting the balance right.

In terms of enhancing health and the development of the immune system, there are other considerations. In choosing a diversity of foods, it is worth considering those which actively provide constituents that help, and avoiding those that have a negative effect.

SUGAR

In order to convert sugars in excess of immediate requirements for storage as fat, the body requires vitamin B. An excessive sugar intake therefore needs lots of vitamin B for this task; vitamin B stores for other uses often become depleted and a deficiency can arise.

We need some sugar, but it occurs naturally in many foods – as fructose in fruit, glucose in honey, and lactose in milk, for example – so sucrose from added sugar and highly-processed foods will provide us with more than we need nutritionally, and can be avoided. Opt for fresh foods whenever you can, avoiding processed foods (which tend to be high in hydrogenated fats and sugars) or pre-prepared foods that have lost much of their nutritional goodness. Eating such foods occasionally won't matter much, but a lot of nutritionally deficient foods, or those high in added sugar, actually sap the body's reserves which could be put to better use.

ORGANIC PRODUCE

Many people are turning more and more to organically produced food, because of anxieties about the use of pesticides, organophosphates, genetically modified food, BSE, etc., and with good reason. However, given that we tend to eat too little fresh produce, perhaps our primary aim in the first instance should be to increase our overall intake of fruit and vegetables. The immediate benefit of this is an important consideration. For many of us, organic produce is becoming more readily available in supermarkets, and it's certainly worth buying, especially root vegetables such as potatoes and carrots. If organic varieties are unavailable, always wash fresh produce carefully and peel off the outer layer.

COOKED OR RAW?

The way in which certain foods are cooked can also increase both their appeal and their nutritional value. Vegetables can be lightly steamed, and many a child who wouldn't touch overcooked carrots at school, and says that he or she hates them, will happily eat them raw or grated, or just cooked.

In fact, some vegetables are better 'just cooked' because if they have a tough, external cellulose wall it's not always easy to get the benefit of their nutritional value when they are eaten raw. A little cooking will soften the cell walls, making their nutrients more digestible.

I tried it every which way, I was so determined to get my child hooked on vegetables and fruit – steamed, puréed, raw – during her first year. And it seemed to work. She's also quite prepared to try things now she's nearly four, and I'm sure it was from constantly trying out all sorts of things to see what she'd like when she was little. Of course, there are some things she just won't eat – celery, for example, partly because of its texture I think, and raw cabbage grated, although she'll eat it cooked.

Tracey, mother to Sara, nearly 4

Vegetables like broccoli, cabbage, or Brussels' sprouts are unappetizing when overcooked, but can be delicious otherwise. Vegetables offered raw are often preferred to those cooked, too. Be flexible in your thinking when it comes to children and food, and diverse in what you offer them, especially when it comes to fruit and vegetables. And if a food is refused outright, don't make an issue out of it, but try offering it again some time later, perhaps prepared or cooked in a different way.

Foods to enhance the immune system

Some foods are thought to positively enhance the immune system, so it's worth introducing these and making them readily available as part of your child's general diet.

APRICOTS

Dried apricots make a delicious snack in themselves, and couldn't be more convenient for a hungry child as you can carry a small packet of them in your bag in readiness. Or you can stew them by bringing them to the boil, simmering them in water for 20 minutes, then serving them whole, or mashed for a baby. Mix with whole-milk yoghurt, ricotta cheese or fromage frais for a complete and nutritious baby meal. Apricots contain beta-carotene, an antioxidant, and are also a good source of iron.

AVOCADOS

Calorie rich, avocados average about 400 calories per fruit. They are also rich in vitamin E and monosaturated fats, plus have useful amounts of vitamins C, D, B_6 and riboflavin. A ripe avocado can be mashed up with ricotta cheese for a baby meal, spread on wholemeal bread for a sandwich for an older child, mashed up into a guacamole dip or added to a mixed salad. They are much more versatile than people think, and one of the best convenience foods around.

BEAN SPROUTS

Beans are already high in vitamin C, but the amount increases by around 600 times once they start sprouting. To retain all this vitamin C content, it is best to eat bean sprouts raw, or perhaps chopped and mixed with other salad items, but they can also be lightly steamed and served cooked in a variety of ways. As a stir-fry ingredient they work well, too.

BEETROOT

This much neglected vegetable has detoxifying properties; it helps to stimulate the liver and the immune system and is a high source of vitamins and minerals. It can be bought ready cooked from the supermarket, but is often available as an organic raw vegetable that is easy to cook (just boil for 15 minutes) or it can be eaten raw, grated into a salad. The leafy tops of beetroot are also edible, contain masses of beta-carotene, calcium and iron, and can be boiled or steamed like spinach. Beetroot is high in natural sugars and is a close vegetable relative to sugar beet, from which we get sucrose. Babies and young children often like the sweetness of the cooked vegetable, which can be mashed or chopped. Raw beetroot juice has quite a strong flavour, but it can be diluted with water or carrot juice to improve the taste for children. Traditionally beetroot has been used as a tonic for convalescents. A word of warning! Beetroot makes the urine quite pink, so don't be surprised by a change of colour!

BLUEBERRIES AND CRANBERRIES

Blueberries are sweeter than many other berries, and can be eaten raw without sugar, providing a source of vitamin C. Research has shown that they also contain antibacterial compounds called anthocyanins, which are effective against some forms of *E. coli*, one of the main culprits of gastroenteritis. Also, like cranberries, blueberries contain a substance that prevents infective bacteria clinging to mucous membranes. For example, recurrent cystitis can be treated by drinking cranberry juice regularly, as bacteria can, literally, be washed away if they are forced to detach from the bladder wall.

Cranberries, however, have a characteristically tart taste and commercially produced cranberry juice contains a lot of added sugar, so be sure to dilute it still further, especially for young children.

GARLIC

Apart from keeping vampires at bay, garlic has wonderful antibacterial and antiviral properties. If you already use onions in your cooking, then you can add garlic too. And if you already use garlic to cook with, use more! For older members of the family there is the additional benefit of garlic's blood-thinning and blood-pressure-lowering properties. And if you are concerned about any residual smell after having eaten it, chew on some fresh parsley, which is rich in vitamin C, too.

GREEN VEGETABLES

Broccoli, spinach and cabbage all contain excellent sources of minerals and vitamins, and the darker green the leaves the higher the source of iron and folates, and folic acid. The trick is to forget your own childhood prejudices about these vegetables, usually horribly overcooked with no nutritional value, and serve them raw or just-cooked, perhaps stir-fried.

NUTS

If you follow a vegetarian diet, and intend your children to do the same, then nuts will form a staple part of their diet. Nuts are high in vitamin E, and a useful source of vitamin B, thiamin and niacin. Small children should never be given nuts in whole form before the age of three, because of the risk of choking, but ground nuts can be used in food preparation quite safely. There is a great deal of concern about peanut allergies, and you may want to check out the use of nuts in your infant's diet with a paediatric nutritionist. Ask your doctor to refer you. The current advice is to not eat large quantities of peanuts during the last three months of pregnancy, as this has been thought to increase the risk of a peanut allergy in young children.

ORANGES

Oranges and other citrus fruits are an excellent source of vitamin C, which is water soluble. Any vitamin C surplus to needs is excreted in the urine as it can't be stored by the body, so it needs to be included in the diet every day. Although juices are high in vitamin C, it is better to eat fresh fruit, which is also a good source of dietary fibre.

Drinks

It is equally important to consider what we give our children to drink, as we can inadvertently counteract some of the benefits of a nutritional diet through what we offer. Drinking water to quench thirst is the best option. Few of us drink enough water, and it is a key requirement, so developing a taste for it and an inclination to drink it in early life is a good thing. But large quantities of any drink can take the edge off an appetite and prevent a child eating an adequate amount of solids. This effect is further exacerbated if the drinks are heavily sweetened. So use soft drinks and fruit juices sparingly, offering water to drink as a first option, or milk if it isn't prior to a meal.

BREASTMILK

Babies who are breastfed need no other drink, although you may want to offer cooled, previously boiled water when the weather's very hot (see below). Breastmilk has a unique ability to adapt to a baby's needs, becoming more watery to quench thirst, as well as being a food supply.

MILK

Give your baby breastmilk, or infant formula, until a year old, although you can use cow's milk in cooking once you've started to introduce solids (and yoghurt and cheese). Whole-fat cow's milk can be given as a drink after a year old, and semi-skimmed milk can be introduced as a drink after two years. Expect your infant or toddler to continue having about a pint of milk a day, in addition to solids, although a proportion of this may be taken in cooking or food sources (custard, yoghurts, etc.). Don't use any sort of unpasteurized milk with infants and children, and avoid goat's and sheep's milk as they are low in folic acid and can mark teeth. Soya milk shouldn't be used except on specific medical advice.

WATER

Cooled, previously boiled water is the best option for a baby to drink. Tap water is fine, but it shouldn't be artificially softened. Bottled mineral waters are not good for babies, the mineral content is far too high and they may also have a bacterial level that is unacceptable for babies. The only acceptable bottled water is Evian. If you use a water filter for tap water, make sure you change it regularly as it can be a good breeding ground for bacteria, and boil filtered water for babies under one year.

> With my first child, I never gave him water – I can't think why now, but I didn't – and now he won't drink it without making a fuss! But I got it right with my second one and introduced cooled, previously boiled water as a drink in a beaker from about four months. And he is always quite happy to have water.
>
> Joanne, mother to Freddy, 6, and Sam, 20 months

SOFT DRINKS

These are notoriously high in sugars and artifical sweeteners and should be restricted to a maximum of two glasses a day, well diluted. Artificially sweetened drinks are not recommended for under-threes. To avoid tooth decay, keep soft drinks to mealtimes only.

FRUIT JUICES

Even natural fruit juices can be high in sugars (fructose) and also high in fruit acids, which can cause damage to your child's milk teeth. Restrict to mealtimes, and dilute as well.

COLAS

Colas and other fizzy drinks are so high in sugar, caffeine and other additives that they shouldn't be given to children under five at all, and should also be restricted to older children. As the occasional treat they are fine, but not as a regular drink.

TEA

Many children are given tea as a drink, though this is mainly a British habit. The tannin binds with any dietary iron available and stops its absorption, so as part of an infant diet tea can be quite detrimental. There is also a tendency to sweeten it with sugar to make it palatable to young children, which provides an unnecessary input of sucrose. Avoid tea as a drink for children, apart from occasionally for older children.

COFFEE

It was recently said that if coffee was discovered today it would be banned as it is so toxic! It's not a popular taste with young children anyway, but for teenagers instant coffee can become a regular habit, and heavily sweetened with sugar, too. As with adults, coffee intake should be limited to a couple of cups a day, at most.

As was said at the beginning of this chapter, while there are very good food choices that can be made, flexibility, diversity and knowledge are key. It is also important not to impose on children the idea that food is either 'good' or 'bad', so that it becomes a source of anxiety – which can only be counter-productive in the long run. Generally, if a few basic principles are adhered to – lots of fruit and vegetables, water to drink, restricted processed foods – then there is always room for the occasional treat. After all, food should be a source of enjoyment as well as nutrients.

5

Boost your child's immune system – Lifestyle

Lifestyle choices

Parents naturally want their child or children to grow up strong and healthy, and will try to provide what is necessary to achieve this. There is no doubt that eating habits and lifestyle choices can have a great influence, and there is also no doubt that promoting positive health should begin early and can be effective. What is also necessary to remember is that while good health in itself won't always prevent illness, it can go a long way to reducing its severity and helping recovery.

Research published in *The Epidemiology of Childhood Disorders* (Oxford University Press, 1994) showed that with few exceptions, for example TB, children's health had little to do with whether or not they actually caught a disease. While malnutrition and the presence of other infections might influence whether or not a child suffered complications from an illness, it didn't actually change the *risk* of getting the illness in the first place.

This theory is borne out in a country like Italy (one of the ten wealthiest nations in the world, and one where you might expect to find a good level of health). But the uptake of whooping cough vaccine is low in Italy and the incidence of the disease relatively high. By law, Italian children must be immunized against diphtheria, tetanus, polio and hepatitis B and show proof of this before they are allowed to attend school. In contrast, the whooping cough and MMR vaccines are only recommended, and currently the whooping cough vaccine uptake stands at around 38 per cent. Epidemics of the disease in Italy tend to occur every three to five years, and around one in four of all Italian children has had whooping cough by his or her fifth birthday. The most severe incidence of whooping cough is in children under the age of one, and in this age group about 1 in 14 babies needs hospitalization, and 1 in 850 dies. In the years between 1980 and 1987, 51 children with whooping cough died and over 80 per cent of these deaths were in babies under the age of one.

Although you cannot remove every risk from your child's life, and whether or not you choose in favour of immunization, it is still worthwhile doing whatever you can to enhance the health of your child. That said, if you can prevent your child getting a secondary bacterial chest infection following a viral cold by providing them with the necessary love, attention, rest and nutrition, this can be very positive.

Providing healthy guidelines

The information provided in Chapters 4–6 provides guidelines on how food, rest, complementary therapies and other aspects of positive lifestyle choices can promote health and the development of a strong immune system.

What we eat is very important (see Chapter 4), as it provides the fuel on which our bodies run. The food we choose to eat is often part of a lifestyle choice, but other aspects of lifestyle are also of importance. The habits learnt in infancy can continue throughout life, and this relates equally to exercise, relaxation, sleep and other lifestyle factors. In supporting those that actively enhance the healthy functioning of the immune system, we can provide our children with healthy guidelines which will continue to influence them throughout their lives. We can provide the foundations on which they can, in the future, base their own lifestyle choices.

In addition to the way we choose to live our lives, there is also an increasing choice of complementary and alternative therapies that can be utilized to good effect, either to encourage positive health or to treat ill-health. More and more parents are turning to these therapies to complement their own, and medical, resources in the care of their children. Descriptions of these therapies, and their application and appropriateness for children, are covered in Chapter 6.

Exercise

Exercise makes an important contribution to a well-functioning immune system, and one of the biggest lifestyle changes for today's children is the lack of naturally occurring exercise. For example, in the 1970s in the UK around 90 per cent of children walked to school each day; now only around 10 per cent do. With physical education no longer a key component of school life, a far less active home life, and limited play areas to roam freely, life is much more sedentary for today's children.

As with all things, balance is the key. It is difficult for younger children to over-exercise, but too little exercise can inhibit the immune system from functioning successfully. However, over-exercising can be a powerful immune suppressor. This may not be an issue now, but during adolescence and a time of rapid growth, excessive exercise can make an individual more, rather than less, prone to every passing infections. Exercise must always be balanced with adequate rest and relaxation. So a degree of television watching is OK, as long as it isn't to the detriment of all physical activity!

Physical exercise is important because the lymphatic system relies on the muscular contractions of the body to keep lymph circulating. Whereas the heart pumps blood around the body, the immune system has no such means of maintaining circulation. It is the lymphatic system that keeps the active cells of the immune system circulating around the body, and physical activity is needed for this to work effectively.

Exercise also has a vital role to play in dispersing the build-up of corticosteroids produced in response to stress, so exercise is a useful antidote. This dispersal of corticosteroids is essential to the functioning of the thymus and lymph nodes, because a continuing excess in the system causes these to shrink, and as a consequence there is a reduction in the production of interferon and T-cells. A reduction in these means the immune system becomes less efficient and less able to respond to and defend the body against infections of various types. For example, this is very obvious after a period of extreme stress, when someone immediately gets a cold. On a more insidious level, a constant degree of low-level stress can keep the immune system functioning below par. And being ill is in itself stressful and demanding of the body. In young children, whose immune systems are still developing, a vicious circle can develop as they seem to catch one infection after another with no respite. This is when it is very useful to look closely at the various ways – improved diet, alternative therapies, more rest – in which you can help restore the good health of your child.

Exercise also has other roles to play: it improves blood circulation generally, so improving both oxygen supply to the body's cells and waste removal from them; it encourages a feeling of wellbeing through the release of endorphins (chemicals in the brain that are released as a result of exercise, and which are natural mood enhancers); and it strengthens the muscles of the heart, improving levels of stamina. Exercise also facilitates fat dispersal and as the lymph is fat-based, keeping fat to an optimum level helps avoid a sluggish system. Children shouldn't be given a low-fat diet, because they need the high calorific content of fat while they are growing and using a lot of energy, but adequate exercise ensures that this doesn't become a problem.

I was getting very concerned about how little exercise my children took, and wondered whether to find some sort of sports club – but that felt like something else that 'had to be done', so I decided that if we just walked to school and back each day, that would be something. No one thought it a good idea at first, because it meant leaving ten minutes earlier than usual. But now it's fine and I don't miss the stress of early morning traffic and trying to find somewhere to park either!

Peter, father to Sally, 9, Luke, 8, and Ross, 6

In children, exercise promotes appetite, and this can be helpful with a child who needs to be encouraged to eat. Exercise also helps them relax and sleep better. Young children have a lot of physical energy that needs channelling if they are expected to sit still for long periods and concentrate – at school, for example. Our bodies were designed for movement, and work better because of it. Not only does exercise influence fat distribution, but it also ensures strong bones. Most importantly, active children tend to continue enjoying activity and become active adults. Overall, because regular exercise is of such enormous benefit in promoting a lifetime's positive health, ensuring our children grow up to be active is very necessary.

Naturally occurring exercise that happens regularly and is part of everyday life can easily be integrated into daily activity with a little thought, and will pay dividends. Allowing five extra minutes to get from A to B, so your child can walk at a natural pace rather than seated in a pushchair or buggy, takes a little extra planning. So often it is quicker and easier to drive somewhere than to walk that it becomes a way of life, and soon the walking option becomes neglected and forgotten.

Light

As well as being beneficial in terms of physical exercise, a daily walk also provides regular exposure to natural daylight. While the dangers of too much sun, especially on young skins, are well known it is also worth remembering that natural light is important for the good functioning of the immune system. Keratinocytes are cells in the skin which produce a substance called interleukin-1 (IL-1). When exposed to natural daylight, the IL-1 in the keratinocytes encourages the production of T-cells, an important part of our immune system.

Exposure to natural daylight doesn't mean sunbathing, just regular opportunities to benefit from natural daylight – which is where the regular walk to school can pay dividends! We are all well aware that we tend to be much healthier and fitter during the summer months, when we can enjoy more outdoor activity. In addition, light is helpful in a type of depression known as SAD (seasonal affective disorder), from which some people, including children, can suffer.

Although strong sunlight can generate oxidants that damage the skin, ensuring a good dietary intake of fresh fruits and vegetables will go a long way to offset this. The judicious use of sunscreens and sunblock for children is essential, but these shouldn't be used on babies under three months old and all babies should be kept out of direct sunlight.

Rest and relaxation

In our increasingly busy lives it is important to remember that children need rest and relaxation in order to recharge their batteries, just as adults do. We seem to live in a culture of constant activity centred around children: after-school activities, play-dates, extra tuition – the list is endless. Some children are entirely happy with this, others find it over-stimulating and too tiring, others just resent never having time to themselves, and yet more cope at some times while not at others. The art of parenting is to try and judge what is right for your child, and respect their wishes if they are expressing discontent or distress in some way.

One winter term, we ended up with so many after-school activities that I spent my time like a constant taxi service. The children always complained about going, although they seemed to enjoy it once they got there, but really I think they just wanted to be at home with their own things. So I cut back drastically: one activity and one play-date a week! It was better, and then as they got older, and in the summer months, we did more.

Gina, mother to Chelsea, 8, and Martin, 6

It is a parent's responsibility to see that children have adequate time off for rest and relaxation, which is particularly important in allowing the body to revitalize itself and support its many systems, including the immune system. Some children find relaxing quite difficult, especially if their environment is very stimulating. Relaxation skills can be learnt, and are of value throughout life and particularly during stressful times. They are also a skill worth learning at an early age.

Quiet times in a child's life may start with the daytime naps of babyhood, through to a rest after lunch, or a quiet storytime before bed. Children need to be given the opportunity to learn how to relish time alone, when they can allow their own thoughts free rein. Children for whom this becomes a pattern in life will seldom complain of boredom: time alone allows them to devise their own occupations, as long as there are facilities close at hand – books, scrap paper, pencils and scissors – for older children to use safely, for example, or an appropriate toy for a younger child. Music and story tapes can also help encourage quiet times, independence and resourcefulness.

When my daughter was 18 months old my mother came to stay, and put together a 'magic box' full of a collection of interesting things – a pine cone, a piece of velvet, a little plastic doll, an exercise book of old photographs of her as a baby, a plastic tea strainer – all sorts of odd things! Then I would leave it near Chloe's cot for the morning. She only had it then. And when she woke she would amuse herself with its contents for an increasingly longer time. It was brilliant for allowing us an extra half hour in the morning, and for Chloe to learn to be happily on her own.

Jill, mother to Chloe, 3

Feeling comfortable alone, or separately within a group, helps a child to learn self-value and can actually help reduce stress now and in years to come. We are all too familiar with the demanding, frenetic, hyperactive child for whom quiet times are too difficult to handle and too threatening to his or her sense of self. Equally, for some children, the constant stress of over-stimulation only serves to aggravate an over-active, or hyper-active, response. This can arise purely from never having been allowed the opportunity to be quietly and comfortably alone. Our physical reaction to over-stimulation and the resultant stress is to produce greater quantities of corticosteroids and adrenaline, which makes us physically jittery and unsettled, as there is often no physical outlet to counteract their effect. Children who are constantly stressed by over-stimulation will show signs of this and often become difficult to manage, while their ability to self-manage their feelings is also impaired.

While it is natural to want to protect children from excess stress, it should also be remembered that many of us thrive on a degree of challenge and stimulation, in the right balance, so it would be wrong to cosset our children so that they never experience stress, or learn to work with and manage it.

Even the secretion of the stress hormone adrenaline has a positive role to play. Recent research has shown that a manageable degree of stressful anticipation helps the body prepare physically, and reduces the impact of physical shock in some instances. So it can be a good thing. This is evident when during a physical crisis – for example, during anaphylactic shock – an injection of adrenaline can be, literally, life saving. As with most things in life, it is a question of balance.

Sleep

The role of sleep in young children's lives is often undervalued. Sleep for many of us is problematic, and as parents we can inadvertently impose our own experience on our children, giving them the idea that peaceful, restorative sleep is difficult to achieve. Very often the first question asked of the parents of a new baby is 'Does he sleep?', because the assumption is that he doesn't! Often there are also assumptions made about a baby being 'good' if he or she sleeps well at night, with the reverse being true if not.

The bottom line is that children need adequate sleep to grow and flourish both physically and emotionally. They also need help in learning how to sleep well. During sleep the two main hormones of wakefulness, corticosteroids and adrenaline, diminish in both secretion levels and activity, which allows other growth hormones to be released. Renewal of body cells also seems to be linked to the body's reduced metabolic rate during sleep, because the cells' reduced oxygen consumption helps to amplify the effects of the growth hormones. Sleep is therefore crucial to the proper functioning of this process and very necessary at times of growth during childhood and adolescence, or during illness.

At birth babies have no diurnal rhythm, i.e. they have no ability to differentiate between day and night — as all new parents are well aware! The development of this ability occurs rapidly as the baby's hormones begin to adapt to light and dark. This is further encouraged by the introduction of routines that outline the day — mealtimes in particular — and bedtime. But of course, the introduction of these gentle, flexible routines takes time to establish.

A baby's sleep requirements are around 15–16 hours a day at four weeks, gradually decreasing until, at the age of two years old, you would expect a toddler to be sleeping for around 12–13 hours a night with at least an hour's nap during the day. Less sleep than this, although feasible, means that the physical demands of growth and activity require some sort of compensation, usually hormonal. An excess of corticosteroids or adrenaline can make a child over-active, fractious and difficult to manage and settle. Many parents say that their babies and young children sleep very little, and don't 'need' as much sleep as others, because they seem so active. This is unlikely to be true, and while it is possible for a child to manage with inadequate sleep, it can be detrimental in the longer term. It can also contribute to an extra demand on the immune system. While a child is well, this may be fine, but at times of additional stress — starting nursery, for example, when there is also exposure to lots of new germs — this may tip the balance towards a run of poor health. Suffice to say that adequate sleep is paramount, and a well-rested child who sleeps well will tend to manage life better.

We expect a lot of our young children: that they should be happy, active and well and also that they should fit in with our lives. The two aren't always immediately compatible and sometimes it becomes imperative to put the physical needs – adequate rest, relaxation and sleep – of a young child first. This is never more obvious than when a child is unwell, and the need for rest and sleep is increased. Hard though it is in our busy lives to consider the idea of fitting in with this demand, it is imperative and will help speed the recovery process and reduce the chance of further opportunistic infections which can attack a compromised immune system. This in turn will help reduce the dependency on you caused by your child's ill-health.

One child psychologist working in an inner-city Child Guidance Clinic once remarked to me that the majority of five-year-olds she saw with behavioural problems were actually suffering from a chronic sleep deficit! So it's worth a thought.

Emotional wellbeing

Some children seem to have been born with a cheerful gene, while others find life troublesome from the start. However, for all children there is much we can do to help them become self-confident and autonomous with a strong sense of self-worth. That journey begins at birth and much of a child's attitude to life will be gleaned from the attitude of those around him or her. Whether or not your child sees a cup as being half full or half empty will depend in part on what your view is of that same cup! The same goes for your attitude to life.

What has also been well established over the years is that emotional wellbeing goes some way in influencing physical wellbeing. As outlined above, stress can play a large part in compromising the successful function of the immune system. How that is dealt with will depend on many factors, including genetic constitution, general health, nutritional status, etc. While a certain amount of stress is inevitable, and positive, it is how or whether we feel able to deal with it that makes a difference. If a potentially stressful situation is perceived as a challenge that can be met, the possible debilitating and daunting aspect of it is reduced. And while some stressful situations are positively relished, there may be an incident that represents the last straw, and which in turn precipitates ill-health.

While we may play lip service to the mind/body link, tangible evidence now shows that high levels of anxiety, depression, hostility and fatigue all result in poor T-cell function. It isn't possible to avoid experiencing negative emotions altogether, but it is possible to learn how to manage both situations and emotions with confidence. Only through time and experience can a child learn that disappointments are inevitable, but manageable; that fear can be overcome, that what was once impossible – climbing to the top of the slide – can become possible and enjoyable.

6

Alternative and complementary therapies

One of the very real benefits of the growing alternative health industry is the increasing availability of properly qualified alternative healthcare practitioners, and in particular those who specialize in caring for children. In addition, more and more health practitioners trained in orthodox medicine are taking on additional training in complementary or alternative therapies in order to extend their professional practice. Many doctors, health visitors, midwives and nurses are now qualifying as homeopaths, acupuncturists, aromatherapists and reflexologists, for example, because they want to provide a useful range of pertinent treatments that are not drug-reliant. And in the area of childcare, these additional skills are often a very useful tool.

Alternative and complementary healthcare is particularly relevant where children's health is concerned for two reasons. First, it provides a resource to actively promote positive health and second, it provides an alternative way of treating many childhood ailments, either on its own or in conjunction with more orthodox treatments. Very often children can suffer some residual complaint, e.g. fatigue following a succession of colds, for which there is no orthodox treatment, but there may be a homeopathic remedy that can alleviate symptoms and aid a fuller recovery. And for eczema that flares up when times are stressful, acupuncture may be a better treatment than steroid creams to relieve a child's symptoms.

As parents we are constantly seeking to protect our children's health, and also to safeguard their future health. As an addition to our parenting skills, knowledge of both the potential and the limitations of alternative and complementary therapies provides an extra resource which we can draw upon when caring for our children. We are all too aware of the problems associated with over-medication, particularly when it comes to the use of antibiotics. Though often an effective resource, and at times life-saving, there are many occasions when antibiotic use is inappropriate. It is of no value in treating viral infections, for example.

When it comes to enhancing a child's developing immune system, there are some very useful alternative resources on which to draw. The purpose of this chapter is to outline these resources and to provide enough information so that parents can make useful choices and extend the opportunities that exist for promoting the positive health of their children.

Homeopathy

A simple description of homeopathy is that it is based on the principle of 'like cures like'. Homeopathy comes from the Greek *homoios* meaning 'like', and *patheia* meaning 'illness'. So a substance which causes the symptoms of a particular illness in a healthy person will, if given in a tiny dose, stimulate the body to produce the response necessary to self-heal the same symptoms in someone who is unwell. This is in contrast to orthodox medicine which tends to use opposites to cure; for example, when treating constipation, laxatives are given.

Because homeopathy works with an individual's energy, both the physical and emotional attitude of a patient have to be taken into account. The mind/body link is integral to wellbeing and how homeopathy works, and as a result there is quite an art to the diagnosis and prescribing of homeopathic remedies. Although there are some remedies that appear to have universal application (Arnica for bruising, for example) the subtlety of homeopathy means that better results always arise from consultation with a skilled and qualified practitioner.

Unlike orthodox medicines, the more dilute the homeopathic dose, the greater its strength, because it has been put through a careful process of potentization. The potency of a remedy is measured as x6, x12, x24 or x30, for example, which refers to the number of times the remedy has been subject to dilution. Homeopathic remedies can be extremely effective; they are also without side effects and have the added benefit of being cheap in comparison to orthodox medicines. Remedies come in a variety of forms, granules, pills, tablets, powders and drops, and they need to be stored away from contaminating substances like peppermint, coffee, eucalyptus oil and other strong, pungent materials. They shouldn't be handled other than by the person for whom the remedy is intended, but instead should be tipped into the lid of the container or onto a clean spoon. The mouth should be clean, i.e. the remedy should not be taken after eating or drinking, and never after drinking coffee or cleaning teeth!

The subtle effectiveness and safety of homeopathy make the remedies a good source of treatment for children, especially as the emotional component of a child's wellbeing is so much a part of their physical disposition. Not only can remedies be prescribed to treat common complaints, they can also be used for their constitutional effect as they can strengthen an individual's ability to deal with distress or illness. And you don't have to believe in homeopathy for it to work; it works on animals just as well!

Homeopathy is sometimes recommended as an alternative to immunization, although homeopaths themselves are not unified in their opinion about this. In the UK, the Faculty of Homeopaths (whose members are trained doctors as well as qualified homeopaths) is unequivocal about recommending immunization: 'We do not have the research data showing the persistence of satisfactory antibody levels after using homeopathic preparations for immunization, and this is why the advice is to use the "conventional" vaccines if at all possible.' The Society of Homeopaths in the UK, whose members are qualified practitioners but not doctors, has no official policy on immunizations but Samuel Hahnemann, the doctor who founded homeopathy in the 18th century, was a strong supporter of it, saying he considered immunization '... a clear and convincing demonstration of the Law of Similitude'.

While there is no evidence to suggest that homeopathy provides long-lasting immunity to an illness, there is enough anecdotal evidence to demonstrate that it can provide some sort of short-term resistance through stimulating the body's natural defences to disease. This probably explains why homeopathy has gained something as a reputation for being an alternative to immunization.

Where there is a known risk from a disease then it is possible to use homeopathic remedies prophylactically to try and prevent contracting the disease. Prophylactic remedies can be a special type of remedy known as a nosode, which is actually made from diseased body tissue or sputum that originally contained the active virus or bacterium. Through the homeopathic process of potentization, these substances become chemically harmless but homeopathically active. For example, if there were an outbreak of whooping cough and your child was unimmunized, you could give regular doses of the nosode Pertussin 30, which studies have shown is beneficial in preventing the disease. However, this would only provide short-term protection and not life-long immunity. Only having the disease, or the vaccination, can provide immunity.

I've always used homeopathy with the children, since they were babies, and consulted a homeopath for specific things. The day Robbie's nursery school teacher told me that one of the other children had gone down with chickenpox, I rang the homeopath who provided me with a remedy to use now and another for when the first spots appeared. I can only say that although it was obvious that he did have chickenpox, it seemed very mild with only a scattering of pustules, none of which got infected. I also gave him a dose of Phenergan [an over-the-counter antihistamine medicine available in the UK] for a couple of nights, so he didn't really suffer from itching and disturbed nights, and the whole illness progressed very smoothly with a fast and full recovery.

Helen, mother to Robbie, 3, and James, 11

There are homeopathic nosodes for all the major illnesses covered by the routine immunizations recommended for young children in the immunization programme, so this does offer the possibility of a protective alternative of sorts, which may be preferred by some parents. However, many alternative practitioners think it is better to get the disease in order to stimulate the immune response and produce the antibodies that should provide life-long protection, rather than avoid this through the use of homeopathic remedies. If you choose to follow this route, there are homeopathic alternatives to nosodes, which will help a child cope better and recover more quickly from symptoms of the disease. For example, you could use Belladonna or Pulsatilla to treat mumps, rather than giving the nosode Parotidinum 30 which might actually prevent the disease. Always consult a qualified and experienced homeopathic practitioner if you want to use homeopathy in this way.

One occasion where the use of homeopathic prophylactic remedies can be invaluable is when travelling. Having first assessed the risks as far as possible, and after discussion with a qualified homeopath, using homeopathic alternatives to travel vaccines may suit many young children better, especially if used alongside other sensible precautions. This is a very specialized area, but one well worth exploring as there is good expertise in this area on which to draw. Ask your homeopath to help you find out all you should consider to travel safely with young children.

Malarial protection is probably one area where very careful consideration should be given. Travelling with children to malarial areas requires careful precautions, which may include orthodox antimalarial treatment as well as homeopathic remedies. Also bear in mind that taking vitamin B yeast seems to make you less attractive to mosquitoes. (Yeast can be taken safely in tablet form by children over the age of five, beginning at least two weeks before and continuing throughout travel.) Or take a tip from the foreign correspondents and eat Marmite or Vegemite! If you can avoid being bitten by following anti-mosquito precautions and using insect repellant you will also avoid such mosquito-borne illnesses as dengue fever as well.

There are, of course, occasions when orthodox medicine should also be brought into play. For example, if a case of meningitis has been diagnosed in a child at the nursery school your child attends, use the homeopathic nosode Meningococcus 30 to help prevent contracting the disease, but at the first sign of any symptoms, seek professional medical advice. A baby or young child's health, and life, could be at risk without proper treatment at a time like this. It doesn't mean, however, that you can't use a variety of alternative and complementary therapies, of which homeopathy would be one, to aid recovery.

It is also thought possible that homeopathic remedies can help the body either to respond more effectively to immunization, or to recover from any side effects from it. One recommendation is to use the homeopathic remedy Thuja 200 before immunization, along with the specific homeopathic preparation for the disease for which immunization is being given; for example, Diphtherinum 200 for diphtheria, and Pertussin 200 for whooping cough. Afterwards, if the vaccination causes a reaction, give the remedy Natrum muriaticum. In this way you can encourage your child's body to react and respond well to immunization, and maximize its benefits. As ever, the benefit of consulting a qualified and experienced homeopath cannot be over-emphasized.

My son had his MMR vaccination at 13 months, and within six hours had spiked a temperature of over 40 degrees Fahrenheit. I stripped him off, gave him infant paracetamol and lots of fluids, but it stayed high for a couple of days. I also rang the homeopath, who immediately prescribed a remedy to counteract the side effects of the vaccine. He was fine, and I felt better knowing I had been able to use homeopathy to help.

Bharti, mother to Arjun, 2

Bach flower remedies

These remedies were developed in the UK in the 1930s by Dr Edward Bach, a conventionally trained and practising doctor who was both a physician and bacteriologist, but who later gave up his Harley Street practice to work as a homeopath. The premise on which Bach based his study and work, and later his remedies, was that the personality of a patient has a profound impact on his or her health, and if you can rebalance or restore emotional health, then this will help restore physical health.

Through his extensive work with plants and their healing properties, Bach originated 38 remedies, including the 'Rescue remedy' which contains a combination of five remedies (Clematis, Cherry Plum, Rock Rose, Impatiens and Star of Bethlehem), and which is designed to provide a source of emotional first aid in the treatment of shock.

The remedies are then subdivided into seven main groups

covering seven emotional states: loneliness, fear, disinterest, oversensitivity, too caring of others, despondency and despair, and uncertainty. Although it is possible to self-treat from the wide range of remedies available, for specific problems a qualified practitioner would be advisable. A careful consultation, balancing the negative aspects of a personality during illness or distress with those that are positive, can give a fuller and more objective picture, leading to a more skilful diagnosis and prescription of the most appropriate remedy, or combination of remedies.

Paediatric osteopathy

Our bodies are made up of interconnecting bones, joints, muscles and ligaments which, ideally, work together and provide a structure to support the internal organs. Our bodies also have a natural inclination to absorb both physical and emotional stress and strain, while attempting always to revert to an internal 'norm', and this requires energy. The body's pull is towards balance, but it cannot always achieve this unassisted, which is why the skills of an osteopath can be very beneficial.

Osteopathy uses manipulation and massage to restore balance in the body's framework, to allow the internal organs the room and opportunity to work most efficiently. The high-velocity thrusts often thought synonymous with osteopathy seldom have a role to play in paediatric osteopathy, which is very gentle and safe.

Most children carry with them some physical effect of their time in the womb, or during labour and birth. And most children can, eventually, find their own balance to adjust to this. But some need a little gentle assistance, if not immediately then perhaps later. It may be that some residual distress is expressed through colic, or sleeplessness or hyperactivity, for example. In any event, the indication for treatment may be very subtle, represented by a minor irritation or grumpiness, which may be deemed as just a part of 'normal' childhood. What these minor irritations may do, however, is draw on energy reserves that could more usefully be used elsewhere. And if there is a more demanding assault on the body's ability to self-regulate its internal balance, perhaps through illness or an accident, then the need for assistance is even greater. Childhood illnesses are part of growing up, allowing the immune system its opportunity to develop antibodies and immunity. Immunization presents another similar opportunity for the production of antibodies. Both events make a physical and emotional demand on the body. These demands can be met and adapted to through the physical support provided by paediatric osteopathy.

> When I took my daughter for an osteopathic check-up, a fortnight after her pre-school booster for DTP and polio, she was fine apart from a little residual tension in the liver. This may not have been connected to the vaccines, or even to a bout of pneumonia which was treated with antibiotics the previous winter, but whatever the reason, and although there were no specific symptoms, I was glad to have it treated.
>
> Ingrid, mother to Sally, 5

Work done in developing paediatric osteopathy in the UK, at the Osteopathic Centre for Children in London, now means that registered osteopaths can embark on a two-year post-graduate training and diploma in paediatric osteopathy. The aim, eventually, is to have these specially qualified osteopaths available to all newly-delivered mothers and their babies to provide a postnatal check. Even babies who have very straightforward births may have been lying awkwardly in the womb. And babies born by Caesarean section, although spared the apparent demands and possible trauma of a vaginal delivery, can be very shocked by their sudden removal from the well-contained internal world of their mother's womb to the outside, and need gentle adjustment to this later.

My first child was born following a high-forceps delivery, with Keilland's forceps used to turn him because of a delay in the second stage. He fed and flourished well, but was a very poor sleeper – still waking every two hours at two years old! Later, we found he had an auditory-perceptual problem which severely affected his literacy skills – learning to read and write was very difficult for him – which was probably as a result of his difficult birth. I just wish I had taken him for paediatric osteopathy after his birth, but I didn't know about it until several years later. My second child had an uneventful birth, and an osteopathic check-up within the first week! They are both very healthy children, and I use homeopathy, massage and paediatric osteopathy – along with immunization and antibiotics – when necessary, but I'm sure my first would have benefited enormously from early osteopathic treatment.

Nicola, mother to Toby, 11, and Alex, 8

When the internal workings of the body are running smoothly and there is harmony between the physical and emotional aspects, then it becomes much easier for children to recover from illness, or to deal with demands like any side effects from immunization, which may be clinically irrelevant but have a subtle effect worth addressing.

Paediatric osteopathy is even gentle enough to use with premature babies, who do in fact benefit enormously from the relief of the stress of their early birth, especially when breathing is restricted or affected by lung immaturity. It releases tensions that may be restricting the correct working of an internal function, and relieves the stress so the body isn't constantly having to compensate for this. An osteopathic check-up at birth can, for many babies, prevent the accumulation of minor stresses that can eventually manifest in tangible symptoms of physical and emotional distress.

Chiropractic

Similar to osteopathy, chiropractic focuses more on the skeletal system and is more concerned with the correct alignment of the spine and joints. This is a treatment of manipulation, and relies on direct pressure and thrusting techniques to diagnose and treat mechanical disorders. Chiropractic has less potential as a therapy for children, and should only be used where the practitioner has specific expertise in treating them. Obviously there is a need to use more gentle techniques, particularly with babies and infants.

Massage and aromatherapy

From the first time you gently stroke your newborn's limbs, to drying your baby after a bath, or playing 'This little piggy...'

with their toes, you are expressing your love and providing security through touch. Massage is a natural progression of this, and one that makes good use of the physical and emotional benefits of positive touch.

Massage can also be used for specific therapeutic effect. Work done at Queen Charlotte's Hospital in London, in the premature baby unit, has shown that massage actually helps to lower the secretion of the stress hormones. Over-production of corticosteroids, as experienced during stressful times, can inhibit both interferon and T-cell production, both important facets of a well-functioning immune system. Massage can also help the circulation of lymph, the transport system of the immune system. So there is a very definite role that massage can play in promoting the development of a strong immune system, and positive health in general.

To massage your baby, infant or child, always use a vegetable-based oil. Avoid baby oils that are petroleum-based, or arachis oils that are derived from peanut oils, and opt for a very light sesame seed or almond oil. It's now possible to find oils specifically designed for use on babies, probably from a specialist alternative supplier, which you can use with confidence.

Always work in a warm, draught-free room, when your baby is alert but peaceful, and neither hungry nor tired. Start with short periods of massage, and if this doesn't seem to suit your baby at the time, stop and try again later. It may be too stimulating and make your baby anxious and fractious, rather than relaxed. It may be that gently massaging your baby's feet is all that can tolerated at first because, while some babies love being massaged from the word go, others find it too demanding and intrusive. Some babies also find having all their clothes removed makes them feel vulnerable, so you may find you need to begin with your baby still wearing a vest, for example. Take your time, and develop a gentle pastime you can both enjoy, using this unique opportunity to communicate with and tune in to your baby.

Use gentle, light finger-tip pressure with just enough firmness to avoid tickling. Start with the feet and gently work up the legs and around the belly in a clockwise direction. Avoid getting too much oil on your baby's hands, especially if you are using essential oils (see below), as babies have a well-known tendency to suck their fingers and rub their eyes. The same applies when gently massaging the scalp and facial area: only use enough oil to allow your hands to move slowly without dragging the skin. Then massage all over the back and buttocks. Remember that a baby massaged with oil is likely to be slippery to hold, so it's often best to place your baby on a soft changing mat and clean towel, on the floor. You can wipe the excess oil off when you wrap your baby in the towel afterwards. Remember, too, that an oily baby can be especially slippery if placed in a bath afterwards, so take care.

In addition to the soothing and therapeutic effects of massaging your baby with oil, you can also use essential oils which provide therapeutic benefits. If using essential oils on babies and children, buy those produced by a reputable supplier and, if you can, opt for oils that have been produced either by steam distillation or expression. Because no solvents or synthetic ingredients have been added to these oils, their purity and potency are undiminished.

Essential oils are potent and effective, so should never be used directly on the skin. Blend with a suitable carrier oil, or a 'white lotion' which can be bought from specialist suppliers of essential oils, or use in water (e.g. added to bath water) or with a vaporizer. All essential oils are antiseptic, some have anti-inflammatory properties, some are healing because they are cicatrizant and help cell regeneration, and others are able to stimulate the immune system. Essential oils are also what is termed 'synergistic', e.g. when several are blended together, the effect of each individual oil is enhanced. This is in part the skill of a qualified and experienced aromatherapist, knowing how to meet a client's needs through the blending of a variety of synergistic essential oils.

The use of massage and essential oils can relieve stress, anxiety or pain in infants and children. The therapeutic properties of the oils permeate the skin and have a subtle physical effect on the body. The smell of different oils can be comforting by association, but in addition they can stimulate the limbic, or emotional, system of the brain, activating good, positive feelings and promoting the release of endorphins which both enhance mood and reduce sensations of pain.

Some essential oils actively stimulate the immune system. For example, tea tree oil helps stimulate the production of T-cells in the blood, the lymphocytes which form the body's first-line response to the presence of viruses, tumour cells and other foreign cells.

Essential oils can also be useful in promoting those abilities to cope with life that help sustain good health. Being able to relax and sleep can be encouraged through the use of oils like camomile, lavender, ylang ylang and sandalwood, for example. Any infection or childhood illness can be debilitating in the long term, and the use of essential oils can help healing and recovery by supporting the body's response to illness and disease, strengthening it and building up its immune response. Numerous very good books exist on the subject (see Further Reading) and the option to consult a qualified practitioner for both treatment and advice in using essential oils at home is well worth considering.

> I took Grace to see an aromatherapist soon after she was born, because I wanted advice about what to use and what use I could make of essential oils for complaints like colic, teething and so on. What I also did when she was three, and had chickenpox, was to consult her again and she made up a massage oil to use. This was a carrier of carrot oil, which has anti-inflammatory properties, plus essential oils of tea tree, geranium and lavender. She also suggested adding bicarbonate of soda to the bath water in addition to the essential oils. Certainly it helped the blisters to heal without scarring and Grace seemed to recover well from the virus, with no after-effects so far.
>
> Maggie, mother to Grace, now 4, and Troy, 14 months

Reflexology

Reflexology is a system of diagnosis and treatment based on the idea that different areas of the foot correspond to specific areas of the body. In this way, massage and manipulation of these specific areas can relieve symptoms. Treatment is very much to do with rebalancing the body's energies, unblocking them and restoring smooth channels of energy between different parts of the body. In this way reflexology is a tool not just for treatment, but also for promoting positive health and stimulating the body's own healing resources.

Reflexology is sometimes referred to as zone therapy, or even compression therapy. Broadly speaking, the right foot corresponds with the right side of the body, and the left with the left. For the purpose of treatment the body is divided into ten vertical channels (or meridians), five on each side, with the energy flowing through these channels from head to toe. By massaging or applying pressure to points on the foot corresponding to the different areas, it is possible to stimulate the nervous and circulatory systems and, by extension, other organs and tissues. Not only is an area massaged, but through manipulation tiny crystals which result from the blockage can be broken down and energy channels revitalized.

Skilled reflexology can be very helpful in treating many childhood ailments, relieving symptoms and enhancing good health. Qualified reflexologists are usually registered with their professional organization. Alternatively, you may find that your doctor or other health professional can recommend one. Check out their experience, and whether they are capable of working with children and happy to do so. Reflexology can be quite potent, so needs to be carried out with care by a practitioner.

Billy was the sort of baby who was born slightly agitated, and found it difficult to feed and settle. It was actually the paediatric osteopath who treated him who recommended some reflexology, and the woman we consulted said there was some tension down his right side (confirmed by the osteopath), which was a residual trauma from a difficult birth. She showed me how to firmly stroke the corresponding area of his right foot, when I massaged his feet with sandalwood oil, and also another spot which relieved intestinal tension, too. It was very helpful to be able to work with these suggestions, and to have an additional way to soothe and settle my baby, knowing it was contributing to his overall health. After about three months he became much more settled, but I still massage his feet before bed. He does love it.

Shelagh, mother to Billy, now 9 months

Many babies and children love having their feet firmly massaged. This isn't the same as reflexology, but more an extension of massage. However, it is worth finding out which areas of the foot might soothe colic or relieve any other form of physical distress that can be a drain on the body's energy resources. You can then gently work around this area yourself. Even the nursery rhyme 'This little piggy went to market …' seems to recognize the benefits to wiggling small people's toes, and massaging the whole foot is very much enjoyed. You can use an essential oil (see above) to increase the benefits, too.

Acupuncture

Traditional Chinese medicine describes the body's energy as flowing through recognizable channels, or meridians, which can get blocked and need stimulating in order to revitalize a particular organ or system of the body. Along the meridians are specific points, at which an acupuncture needle can be inserted to provide the stimulation necessary. This energy is referred to as 'Chi' (pronounced *chee*), and is governed by the inseparable but opposite forces of yin (masculine) and yang (feminine). For the body to work harmoniously, these two forces have to be in balance, otherwise illness or physical distress will occur.

An acupuncturist who treats children needs to have specialist experience in this area, and may have undergone additional training. Instead of using the very fine sterile disposable needles, the acupuncturist will use finger-tip pressure (see Acupressure, below). Treatment can be used to help relieve symptoms; for example, it has been shown to be effective with both allergies and asthma. Acupuncture is also useful for pain relief as it stimulates the production of endorphins. And any treatment that enables the body to rebalance and to focus internal energy on developing good health leaves the body free, in a sense, to get on with the important task of developing a strong immune system.

Acupressure

Using the same system of energy channels, or meridians, described above, finger-tip pressure rather than needles is applied to specific points along the meridians. The Japanese system of acupressure is called Shiatsu, but all three systems work on the principle of restoring energy flow, rebalancing the body, relieving symptoms and enhancing positive health. Allowing the body to utilize its own self-healing mechanisms, and supporting it in this task with treatments like acupressure, can be extremely useful in ensuring recovery from any physical or emotional assault on the body resulting from illness or a period of poor health.

Naturopathy

This is a term that describes a multifaceted approach to promoting health and treating illness. In much the same way that Traditional Chinese medicine might incorporate acupuncture, herbal medicine, t'ai chi and a particular philosophy about the causes of poor health and disease, so it is with naturopathy.

The aim of naturopathy is to restore and maintain health by giving the body what it needs to function properly, through a nutritious wholefood diet, adequate exercise, rest and relaxation, a positive mental attitude, fresh air and an unpolluted atmosphere – all of which will strengthen the immune function of the body and enhance the ability to self-heal.

In specific application, naturopathy is quite rigorous, but for many of us its aims are incorporated to a degree in the way in which we try to raise our children within a healthy lifestyle. This is appropriate because many naturopaths see themselves as teachers, helping individuals to learn what they need in order to take responsibility for their own lives. As long as balance exists, the body is capable of functioning well enough to fight off invading organisms and self-heal. And this balance can be reinforced by good nutrition, vitamin and mineral supplements where indicated, breathing exercises, physical exercise, and herbal or homeopathic medicines where appropriate. Naturopathic therapy also includes fasting, massage and hydrotherapy, while it is likely that any naturopath you consult will have training in osteopathy, too.

Consulting a naturopath can be very useful in addressing a

specific health issue in a child, or for assessing how lifestyle changes might be valuable in developing a strong immune system and good health in general. Learning how to boost the body's own defence systems, through diet for example, can be extremely beneficial not just during childhood, but throughout life. Understanding how the body is able to deal with illness, through fever or inflammation, for example, and how these processes need to be allowed to happen, lies at the heart of naturopathic philosophy. So continual promotion of positive health, in all its forms, is essential in supporting the body and enabling it to function properly.

We consulted a naturopath because Miriam had had continuous poor health – in the form of endless coughs, colds and ear infections – from the age of about two. We introduced a wholefood diet, with organic foods where we could manage it, but lots more fruit and vegetables and no processed foods at all. We also cut out wheat products. She was prescribed homeopathic remedies and had some osteopathy. Also, we started swimming every week which helped open up her chest and improved her breathing. All of which contributed to a calmer child, who relaxed more easily and slept much better. After a year not only were there no more endless colds and chest infections, but she was much stronger, fitter and able to cope with life much better. We put off sending her to nursery until she was four, just to be sure she could cope. Now, at almost six, she is a picture of positive health and we just check in with the naturopath every six months. He also gave us advice when her sister was born.

Peter, father to Miriam, 6, and Rebecca, 11 months

Applied kinesiology

Kinesiology is a diagnostic system which assesses the strength of a muscle (which can vary considerably) when an individual is exposed to a substance to which the body is sensitive or intolerant. It was in the 1960s that an American doctor and chiropractor, Dr George Goodheart, who was using kinesiology as a diagnostic tool, discovered a link between patients' muscle strength and tone and the state of their internal organs. He found that by applying what he had diagnosed with kinesiology, and using firm pressure on areas of muscle, he could rebalance the energy flow and relieve symptoms of specific illness or physical distress.

Since then, the practice of applied kinesiology has developed and practitioners have to be properly trained and qualified, usually holding a diploma, which in the UK is the Diploma of the Association of Systematic Kinesiology (DipASK). Treatment is through the revitalization of energy in the muscles, and may be carried out in combination with chiropractic or other physical therapies. Advice on diet and the use of vitamin or mineral supplements may also be given.

Often kinesiologists are consulted to identify food intolerance, for example lactose intolerance, which may be the cause of other symptoms or disorders in the body. As with all alternative therapies, the practitioner has to be experienced in its application to infants and children, and may make modifications in treatment practice to accommodate this. Again, this therapy may be used to treat specific ailments, for example chickenpox, or it may be a useful resource to maintain good health and allow the body to function to its full capacity.

Alternative and complementary therapies

Herbal medicine

Plants have a unique energy that can be used to help the body's natural ability to rebalance and self-heal. Specific plants have specific properties that can be used, and herbal medicines and remedies – using the whole plant in their preparation – harness the plant's energy for our use. These preparations come in numerous forms – decoctions, infusions or tinctures, for example – but can also be prepared as compresses, ointments or syrups. In contrast, conventional drugs, even when the original source is a natural one, isolate the chemical component rather than utilizing all the plant's components and, as a consequence, its energy.

As with other complementary therapies and remedies, the aim of treatment is not just to treat disease and poor health, but also to actively create a balance in the body and help prevent illness. Plant medicines, or herbal remedies, can be extremely potent and should only be prescribed by a qualified herbal practitioner. In the UK, the National Institute of Medical Herbalists (NIMH) registers those herbalists who have completed the required training to qualify. A practitioner with the initials MNIMH is a member of the National Institute, and with FNIMH is a fellow.

Herbal medicine can be very useful in helping the strong development of the immune system in a child. It can also be used to treat illness, aid recovery and convalescence, and as an antidote to the side effects of some orthodox treatments, like antibiotics. One herb that many of us eat regularly is garlic, which has exceptional properties and is one of nature's most reliant antimicrobial resources, effective against bacterial, viral and fungal organisms.

Other familiar herbs include echinacea and ginseng, well known for their ability to strengthen and enhance the body's immune response. Echinacea is also known by the names purple cornflower, Missouri snakeroot and black samson. It is native to North America, where the North American indians have used it traditionally for centuries. It is one of the best herbs for helping the body fight infections because it helps cleanse the blood, has a stimulating effect on the immune system and activates white blood cells and antibodies. It also speeds healing and reduces inflammation. In specially prepared form it is taken by mouth, but can also be used externally as a wash for eczema, sores, cuts and bites. It does, however, work best in the short-term and should only be used during acute infection for around five to seven days, after which it should be discontinued for three or four days, before starting again if necessary. Echinacea shouldn't be taken every day, and is useful as a precaution rather than a healing substance.

Ginseng is also able to boost immunity. However, it shouldn't be taken during active illness, but following infection or to promote positive health as a tonic. It is known to help increase the white blood cell count in convalescing patients, and also helps the liver and spleen in both their detoxification and immunological activities.

Other herbs that are useful for promoting the efficient functioning of the immune system are astragalus, burdock and dandelion. Often the root of these herbs is used, and in combination can create a beneficial tonic for promoting good health and helping the body detoxify, keeping its systems functioning well.

Numerous other herbs are useful for helping children recover from infection and, as always, the advice of a medical herbalist is invaluable. These herbs include camomile, eyebright, catnip, goldenseal, liquorice, slippery elm and ginger. Because herbs can be extremely potent, they need to be administered with caution and only given in therapeutic doses when prescribed by a qualified medical herbalist.

Although I've used herbal remedies, bought from the local health store, for the children it wasn't until Lia had a nasty bout of chickenpox, followed by a chest infection, that I consulted a medical herbalist. I wanted to find some sort of tonic that was specific, that would help Lia get over a viral infection followed by a bacterial infection, followed by treatment with antibiotics. This had left her feeling very washed out, lethargic and depressed – not like my usually bouncy seven-year-old! She was prescribed a combination of goldenseal, dandelion and echinacea for five days, followed by Chinese angelica and ginseng for a further week. I was also advised to let her rest more, and give her lots of fresh fruit and vegetables – organic where possible. After about four weeks she was greatly recovered, and managed to get through the rest of the winter without even a cold!

Shona, mother to Lia, 7, Tom, 3, and Caitlin, 9 months

Chinese herbalism

Herbalism is a part of Traditional Chinese medicine, which also includes acupuncture (see above). Like the majority of alternative practices, and acupuncture in particular, the aim of Chinese herbalism is to treat the individual not the illness, ailment or disease – which are the symptoms specific to the individual. Again, because of the potency of the herbs used, it is essential to consult a qualified practitioner. It is also imperative that anything prescribed for one person isn't given to anyone else. Under the correct conditions, Chinese herbalism is safe and effective, and many complaints respond well to treatment. These include skin problems (for example, eczema, psoriasis, and acne), hay fever, period problems, anaemia and viral infections. Stress, too, can be helped. Chinese herbs given as a tonic can be helpful in recovering from the stress of an infection, allowing the body to rebalance and for its systems to function with greater strength.

Meditation

There is no doubt that meditation, if properly practised, can have a profound effect on the physical functioning of the body. It has been described as '... a state of poised, highly directed concentration, focused not upon a train of thoughts or ideas, but upon a single, clearly defined stimulus' (*Teaching Meditation to Children*, by Dr David Fontana and Ingrid Slack). Among the many well-known benefits of meditation are physical relaxation, stress reduction, and improved concentration and memory. By affecting the emotional state of an individual positively, it is possible for the internal, physical workings of the body to benefit. Meditation has also been shown to improve the functioning and number of T-cells and lymphocytes, thus contributing to a well-functioning and efficient immune system.

But can it, and should it, be taught to children? The short answer is that if children are taught the skills of meditation from an early age, they have a resource of enormous value available to them throughout their lives. However, it should also be said that because children are open and impressionable by nature – which in part is why meditation and relaxation skills can be very easy to teach to children – then any teaching of this type should be provided without any suggestion of religious or cultish overtones. And there is no reason why this shouldn't be possible: meditation is a skill like any other. The aim is to give children power and control over their thoughts and emotions, not through self-repression but through greater self-awareness and self-acceptance. And providing a child with a sense of self-management goes a long way to providing the autonomony that makes what life throws at us more manageable, which in turn reduces how stressful we may find it.

Before the age of about five, it is difficult to teach meditative skills but the preparatory work – learning to be still, to listen, to be peacefully quiet – can begin. What can be focused on from around the age of five are some of the physical processes that lead towards a meditative state. Starting with breathing, and an observation of breathing in and out, helps begin the concentration necessary to reduce the distraction of thoughts as they arise. Using a mantra, or a phrase such as 'I am happy', repeated softly on each out breath, reinforces this focus. This is also an opportunity to reinforce the positive.

Childhood is, by its nature, an emotional time. Everything from happiness to anger is felt much more acutely, and emotions can be very powerful and even frightening. Learning to understand emotions is part of the journey of childhood, and emotions like fear and anger can be overwhelming, literally, to a small person. The process of learning meditation skills inevitably focuses on emotions, and this opportunity to do so can be a way of helping children to acknowledge, and master these big feelings, and to accept them rather than repress them. Repressing big feelings is seldom helpful, and living with unreconciled feelings creates a continuous stress that places unnecessary burdens on the physical body.

To become fully able to meditate, children need proper teaching. Check out what is available locally, attend yourself, and ensure you are happy with what is being taught. Ask about special children's classes; they may perhaps be described as relaxation classes or exist as an adjunct to a children's yoga class.

I have meditated for years; it began as a continuation of a yoga course I began in pregnancy and I found it very helpful during early parenthood. I was keen for the children to learn, eventually, although because it was something I did, they thought it was very un-cool! But we had always massaged them when babies, and encouraged deep breathing and relaxation, so when my eldest, Beccy, was becoming quite competitive with her swimming, aged about 10, I had suggested that it might be a helpful way to prevent nervousness before competitions. She also understood that because breathing is so important to swimming, this might be useful too. More importantly, perhaps, her coach agreed with the idea. Then I found someone who taught children, and who was very un-flaky and knew how to roller blade, which impressed the kids! I was very pleased, not so much for Beccy but for her younger brother, Sean. He has always been quite moody and easily frustrated if things don't go his way, and it's helped him enormously.

Sylvia, mother to Beccy, now 12, and Sean, 9

T'ai chi

This form of Chinese exercise is worth a mention here because it is, essentially, meditation in motion. Because of this, many children find the idea of meditation in this way more acceptable, although in the view of most teachers it isn't suitable for children under the age of 10.

Through physical activity, the aim of t'ai chi is to create harmony within the body which can then have an effect at a spiritual and emotional level. This in turn develops an inner life, activating the life force, or chi, making it available for rebalancing and healing the body when necessary. Once learnt, t'ai chi is extremely effective at reducing stress and revitalising energy sources.

T'ai chi needs to be taught by a skilled practitioner who has a teaching diploma and at least 10 years' experience, including studying with a master. Although serious in intent, classes for children need to be enjoyable and focused, otherwise the children become bored and inattentive. If the class is so large that a child needs to be completely self-reliant in order to learn, this will probably be counter-productive.

T'ai chi is suitable for children of all levels of physical ability because there is no competitive element: it provides a degree of exercise, but more importantly it focuses the mind through body movements and the only aim is to find the still, internal place which calms and revitalizes the body and mind allowing the body systems to function with greater efficiency.

Paul was diagnosed with dyspraxia, eventually, when he was 12. Although good to have a diagnosis, there's not much practical assistance offered so we looked at what alternative and complementary approaches we could take, and because there was a good t'ai chi teacher in our area, we considered this and I spoke to the teacher about it. We agreed that this might be beneficial, and it has proved to be wonderfully helpful although Paul found it very difficult at first. And it's been good for me too, because I've been doing classes as well, with him, and my blood pressure has come right back down to normal!

Graeme, father to Paul, now 16

Yoga

Yoga for children is becoming increasingly popular, and with good reason. Not only is it a non-competitive form of physical exercise, it also encourages good posture and better breathing, concentration, self-awareness, stress management and relaxation. It teaches children how to use their bodies, maintaining flexibility, and how to be still. It is also effective in helping with problems like asthma, insomnia, headaches and constipation. And in general terms, yoga helps the body get rid of toxins, enabling its systems to function effectively.

In addition, yoga is fun and can help engender a sense of self-confidence, because for many children yoga is easy compared to other forms of exercise, which can often be competitive and at which few children excel. It is also something in which the whole family can join, and something that can be practised at home. Often parents who practise at home find their young children, quite spontaneously, joining in. So it's possible to introduce yoga from a relatively young age. Certainly it is seldom too young to introduce the idea of doing something peacefully alone, and for its own sake, especially when the return is an inner sense of composure.

Appendix

US immunization schedule

Recommended Childhood Immunization Schedule United States, January – December 1999

Vaccines are listed under routinely recommended ages.

Bars indicate range of recommended ages for immunization.

Age ▶ Vaccine ▼	Birth	1 mo	2 mos	4 mos	6 mos	12 mos
Hepatitis B		Hepatitis B				
			Hepatitis B		Hepatitis B	
Diphtheria, Tetanus, Pertussis			DTP	DTP	DTP	
H. influenzae type b			Hib	Hib	Hib	Hib
Polio			IPV	IPV	Polio	
Rotavirus			Rv	Rv	Rv	
Measles, Mumps, Rubella						MMR
Varicella						Var

Any dose not given at the recommended age should be given as a "catch-up" immunization at any subsequent visit when indicated as feasible. Ovals indicate vaccines to be given if previously recommended doses were missed or given earlier than the recommended minimum age.

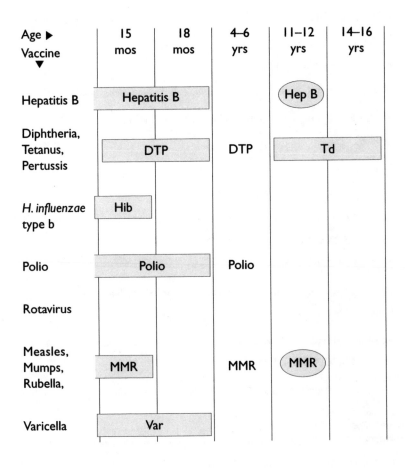

Age ▶ Vaccine ▼	15 mos	18 mos	4–6 yrs	11–12 yrs	14–16 yrs
Hepatitis B	Hepatitis B			Hep B	
Diphtheria, Tetanus, Pertussis		DTP	DTP	Td	
H. influenzae type b	Hib				
Polio		Polio	Polio		
Rotavirus					
Measles, Mumps, Rubella,	MMR		MMR	MMR	
Varicella		Var			

Further Reading

Bedford, Helen, and **David Elliman,** *Childhood Immunisation: A review for parents and carers,* Health Education Authority, London, 1998.

Bove, Mary, *An Encyclopedia of Natural Healing for Children and Infants,* Keats Publishing, Connecticut, 1995.

Burney, Lucy, *Optimum Nutrition for Babies and Young Children,* Piatkus Books, London, 1999.

Castro, Miranda, *Homeopathy for Mother and Baby,* Pan Books, London, 1992.

McIntyre, Anne, *The Herbal for Mother and Child,* Element Books, Shaftesbury, 1992.

McTaggart, Lynne (ed), *My Healthy Child,* The Wallace Press, London, 1997.

McTaggart, Lynne (ed), *The Vaccination Bible,* The Wallace Press, London, 1997.

Meek, Jennifer, and **Patrick Holford,** *Boost Your Immune System,* Piatkus Books, London, 1998.

Natural Parent (magazine published six times a year), 77 Grosvenor Avenue, London N5 2NN. Tel: 020 7354 4592
E-mail: wddty@zoo.co.uk

Price, Shirley, and **Penny Price Parr,** *Aromatherapy for Babies and Children,* Thorsons, London, 1996.

Salisbury, David, and **Norman Begg** (eds), *Immunisation Against Infectious Disease,* HMSO, London, 1996.

Sharma, Dr R., *The Element Family Encyclopedia of Health,* Element Books, Shaftesbury, 1998.

Sinclair, Ian, *The Alternative to Vaccination: Health, the Only Immunity,* Ian Sinclair Publications, Australia, 1995.

Useful Addresses

UNITED KINGDOM

Association of Breastfeeding Mothers

PO Box 207

Bridgwater

Somerset TA6 7YT

Tel: 01727 859 189

Association of Parents of Vaccine Damaged Children

2 Church Street

Shipston on Stour

Warwickshire CV36 4AP

Tel: 01608 661595

British College of Naturopathy & Osteopathy

3 Sumpter Close

120–122 Finchley Road

London NW3 5HR

Tel: 020 7435 6464

British Acupuncture Council

Park House

206–208 Latimer Road

London W10 6RE

Tel: 020 8964 0222

British Homeopathic Association

27a Devonshire Street

London W1N 1RJ

Tel: 020 7935 2163

Dr Edward Bach Centre

Mount Vernon

Sotwell

Wallingford

Oxon OX10 0PZ

Tel: 01491 834678

General Council & Register of Naturopaths

Goswell House

2 Goswell Road

Street

Somerset BA16 0JG

Tel: 01458 840072

Health Education Authority

Trevelyn House

30 Great Peter Street

London SW1P 2HW

Tel: 020 7222 5300

The Informed Parent

PO Box 870

Harrow

Middlesex HA3 7UW

Tel: 020 8861 1022

Institute of Optimum Nutrition

Blades Court

Dodar Road

London SW15 2MU

Tel: 020 8877 9993

International Federation of Aromatherapists
Stanford House
Chiswick High Road
London W4 1TH
Tel: 020 8742 2605

JABS (Justice, Awareness & Basic Support)
1 Gawsworth Road
Golborne
Warrington WA3 3RF
Tel: 01942 713565

La Leche League
BM 3424
London WC1N 3XX
Tel: 020 7242 1278

Medical Advisory Service for Travellers Abroad (MASTA)
London School of Hygiene and Tropical Medicine
Keppel Street
London WC1E 7HT
Tel: 09068 224 100

National Institute of Medical Herbalists
56 Longbrook Street
Exeter
Devon EX4 6AH
Tel: 01392 426022

Osteopathic Centre for Children
109 Harley Street
London W1N 1DG
Tel: 020 7486 6160

Vaccination Awareness Network UK

178 Mansfield Road

Nottingham NG1 3HW

Tel: 0115 948 0829

What the Doctors Don't Tell You

4 Wallace Road

London N1 2PG

Tel: 020 7354 4592

E-mail: wddty@zoo.co.uk

USA

American Association of Acupuncture and Oriental Medicine

1424 16th Street NW

Suite 501

Washington DC 20036

American Aromatherapy Association

PO Box 3679

South Pasadena

CA 94903

American Academy of Paediatrics

141 Northwest Point Boulevard

Elk Grove Village

IL 60007–1098

Tel: 847 228 5005

American Osteopathic Association

142 East Ohio Street

Chicago

IL 60611

Tel: 312 280 5800

American Herbalists Guild

PO Box 1683

Sequel

CA 95073

Tel: 408 484 2441

American Holistic Medical Association

4101 Lake Boone Trail

Suite 201

Raleigh

NC 27607

Tel: 919 787 5181

American Institute of Homeopathy

1585 Glencoe

Denver

CO 80220

Tel: 303 370 9164

Dr Edward Bach Healing Society

644 Merrick Road

Lynbrook

NY 11598

Tel: 516 593 2206

La Leche League International

PO Box 1209

Franklin Park

IL 60131–8209

Homeopathic Academy of Naturopathic Physicians

PO Box 69565

Portland

OR 97201

Tel: 503 795 0579

International Association of Infant Massage

PO Box 438

Elma

NY 14059-0438

Tel: 716 652 9789

American Naturopathic Association

1413 King Street

First Floor

Washington

DC 20005

Tel: 202 682 7352

A*USTRALIA*

Acupuncture Ethics & Standards Organisation

PO Box 84

Merrylands

NSW

Tel: 0061 296 827882

Australian College of Alternative Medicine

11 Howard Avenue

Mount Waverley

Victoria 3149

Australian College of Nutritional and Environmental Medicine

13 Hilton Road

Beamaris

Victoria 3193

Tel: 03 9589 6088

Australian Federation of Homeopaths

238 Ballarat Road

Footscray

Victoria 3011

Tel: 03 9318 3057

Australian Natural Therapists Association

PO Box 308

Melrose Park

South Australia 5039

Tel: 618 297 9533

Australian Osteopathy Association
PO Box 699
Turramurra
NSW 2074
Tel: 02 449 4799

Australian Traditional Medicine Society
Suite Three, First Floor
120 Blaxendle Road
Ryde, NSW 2112
Tel: 612 808 2825

International Federation of Aromatherapists
1/390 Burwood Road
Hawthorn
BIC 3122
Tel: 03 9530 0067

National Herbalists Association of Australia
Suite 305, BST House
Small Street, Broadway
NSW 2007
Tel: 02 211 6437

Nursing Mothers Association of Australia
16 Dinsdale Place
Hamersley
WA 6022

Index